Ho

M000015271

R.A.I.S.E.
an Athlete
The Formula

By Renowned Orthopedic
Surgeon to the Athletes
Dr. Richard C. Lehman
with Cameron Lehman

How To R.A.I.S.E. An Athlete – The Formula
Author: Lehman, Richard C., Dr.

Contributing Editor: Lehman, Cameron

Cover Design: Altaris Design
Interior Layout: Romans 12:21 Creation

Bulk orders available for distribution through IngramSpark or requested by emailing RaiseAthleteIQ@gmail.com.

ISBN-10: 1736541NaN
ISBN-13: 978-1736541005

Printed in the United States of America

Advanced Praise

"From the first time we met, I realized Doc knew his stuff. He was caring and thought about ME, long term, and beyond the competition. It wasn't just about how we could get the athlete better and faster. It was a relationship and it just grew from there. He's part of the team."

Jackie Joyner-Kersee
Sports Illustrated's
Greatest Female Athlete Of The Twentieth Century
Track and Field Four-Time Olympian and
Seven-Time Medalist

"Rick is a dedicated surgeon who has done all he could to facilitate and extend the careers of so many players. His legacy is how he integrated his knowledge of so many sports into treatment methods for so many athletes. He is on the cutting edge of sports medicine."

"Iron" Mike Keenan
Stanley Cup Winning NHL Coach

"It does the doc a disservice to put a definition to who he is, but I'll try. He is a consummate loving professional and, in my opinion (and many others'), the greatest orthopedic surgeon on this earth."

Nino Fennoy
Track & Field Coach
Mentor to Generations of Olympians

"With Rick, it's about them, the patients. It's about their whole life. It's all about delivery. It's a team effort. He works with people who understand that."

Carla Droege
X-Ray Specialist and Medical Professional
Long-time Partner to Dr. Lehman

"Rick is so personable and down to Earth. I love the good doctor's sense of humor. Dr. Lehman always puts the players' interests above the team and league interests. Rick's bedside manner far exceeds that of so many other (if not all other) surgeons and his self-deprecating sense of humor separates him from others as a surgeon and as a person. With Dr. Lehman, the athlete always comes first."

Rob Campbell
NHL Coach

"I have three Division 1 athletes in my family: two sons and a daughter. I was referred to Dr. Lehman and he would get them in the best possible shape. Everything creative and aggressive, but still safe, Doc and his team do. As a Dad of three athletes and a lover of sports, I enjoy more than anything how he takes care of his patients, sometimes MY kids, as his NUMBER ONE priority. Always. When my daughter moved away as an adult and was training for a marathon, I remember her calling me and saying, 'I miss Dr. Lehman.' He is so much a part of what made my family successful in sports and healthy for life at the same time."

Frank Cusumano
Sportscaster (KSDK), Father, Husband, and Believer
Missouri Sports Hall of Fame

"He is one of the best doctors, or THE BEST probably, I've ever worked with in all of sports. Football, hockey, track and field, tennis, basketball . . . you name it! If I ever had a problem or injury, he is the first one I call. And not just in orthopedics. He knows the whole body, knows the best people to help when it's not him, and loves people enough to take care of them no matter what."

Bobby Kersee
Most Winning Olympic Track and Field
Coach in U.S. History

Table of Contents

Dedicated to

the COVID-19

pandemic athletes.

Many of you lost your seasons;
may this book help you have many more.

The Do-Over

When Coronavirus shut down NBA Basketball, then NHL Hockey, then NCAA sports, then high school sports around the country, and then Major League Baseball (MLB) was delayed indefinitely . . . ultimately followed by all of the other major professional sports around the country and internationally—including the 2020 Summer Olympics in Tokyo—the world I work in became, as for everybody, very unfamiliar. News and the internet remained full of daily statistics and briefings presented with newscasters socially distanced, one of many terms that have become part of our daily language; spotlights were moved from our celebrities and athletes to hardworking colleagues of mine in medicine; and we started to recognize and appreciate the workers bearing our daily life essentials such as groceries, home entertainment, and maintenance items—all while our homes, themselves, became schools, offices, playgrounds, and hobby shops.

It's true some long overdue praise was heaped on our essential workers, but I believe we also grew a new gratitude for athletics in an "absence makes the heart grow fonder" sort of way. I just love sports and not just pro sports. I love college sports. I love seeing high school athletes who take that next step toward Division I sports. As fun as it is watching the development of those I've cared for, I really do love the sports. And this season has highlighted a similar love in others.

We miss the bonding with whole communities of strangers over shared team allegiances, the frenetic cheering on of our players, and the excitement of gathering in crowded sports venues (those in the fresh air and those indoors and filled with the scents of sports flooring and stadium foods). It's surreal how strange those scenes now seem. We also miss the sports, themselves—the inspiring displays of physical aptitude, strength, and agility wrestling it out with all they have for the glory of the moment. Our priorities may have shifted, but our love of the game has merely marinated, growing in flavor and desire as we await the return of our athletic heroes.

> *Our priorities may have shifted, but our love of the game has merely marinated, growing in flavor and desire as we await the return of our athletic heroes.*

We're almost a year past those first shutdowns of the pandemic and, through the miracle of science, the worldwide vaccination effort is under way. When this is all a memory in our post-COVID-19 world, I think we'll need sports more than ever. We'll need to come together again after our world has been torn apart and sports is one of the few things that allow that human connection. We don't have to share political views or backgrounds to share in the love of athletics. We'll need the contrast of simple pastimes and fanatical jubilance that comes from sports. There are some valuable lessons that will no doubt come out of this unprecedented season, but the games will return and, therefore, so will our athletes.

Maybe we can do it better if—in our reset—we take on some new knowledge of how we raise our athletes. In fact, I think we're obligated to do better! Let's take care of our athletes, our young people, in a way that sets realistic expectations, manages their overall and wholistic health, and prepares them for life beyond the courts and fields of play to the years they have after they hang up their athletic shoes.

The knowledge of how we raise our athletes is just as important now as it has ever been. Maybe more, because—while nobody asked for it—we have an opportunity for the ultimate athletic gift: a do-over.

Let's not screw this up!

The Greatest

While my friendship with the famous track and field coach went back further, I'll never forget a shared moment with Bobby Kersee during the 1996 Olympics in Atlanta. Rain was in the air, but the events went on, including the heptathlon, an event that Bobby's wife Jackie Joyner-Kersee had dominated in Olympics, World Championships, Goodwill Games, and the record books for nearly two decades. (At the time of this printing, she still holds the world record in that event, along with the next six all-time best results, in a long list of other athletic achievements.) After injuring her hamstring in the qualifying rounds, the incredibly taxing 100-Meter Hurdle event was going to be grueling, but Jackie was a competitor, so her will and her training would have to carry her more than her muscles in the race.

Bobby and I closely watched her in the third heat, observing every stride Jackie took. Before the halfway point, and with a concentrated strain on her face, Jackie had already solidified a significant lead. The white tape holding her hamstring firm served as another visible manifestation of her pain. While she maintained her lead throughout the 13.26 seconds that felt like days, by hurdles nine and 10, she was struggling. I cringed watching her leap over the final hurdle. Jackie's favoring of her strong leg resulted in an almost lopsided landing as she cleared the obstacle. She pushed through the final two strides, leaned her body forward to gain inches with her long frame, and crossed the finish line in first, as few but Jackie knew how to do. Her face collapsed excruciatingly, and she breathed heavily, not from the exertion as much from what was clearly physical anguish.

On televisions in homes we couldn't be in, one reporter was quoted as saying, "I think that could be the end of what we would almost consider the greatest ever female athlete." (Sports Illustrated actually named her the *"Greatest Female Athlete Of The Twentieth Century."*)

Bobby and I shared a look that said what we didn't need to speak out loud: Jackie might be done. Bobby rushed to her, me right alongside him. Jackie voiced that she wanted to continue and look toward the high jump. She was pushing. She was a champion. Jackie would have been willing to injure every muscle in her body for this one more championship. And that's when Bobby the coach stepped back and let Bobby the husband step in.

"I'm not gonna let you do this," he said.

"I want to try," Jackie returned.

Bobby cried. Jackie cried. The world's cameras were on them while one of its greatest-ever athletes felt as though her final medal was slipping away. Bobby literally carried Jackie off the track.

All eyes were on Bobby, Jackie, and I. This was a gut-wrenching moment in sports history.

An athlete will always choose momentary triumph over the potential reality of long-term impairment. Glory is their nourishment. That's where families, coaches, and doctors come in. Jackie needed to heal and, finally, she surrendered to that decision. He convinced her to walk away. Olympic history was happening before our eyes. Bobby was ready to go home entirely, but the compromise was to spend the time getting Jackie healed and prepared to compete in the long jump, the last and Jackie's favorite part of the heptathlon.

We had five days to build a comeback story.

◆ ◆ ◆ ◆ ◆ ◆

Maybe I should start at the beginning. I grew up with a modest family in Miami and, from an early age, I loved sports and competition. I especially had a great appreciation for tennis. As the competition grew, so did my love for the sport, and I became an accomplished player. I aspired to professional athletics and truly believed tennis was going to get me there.

I attended Miami Norland High School. It was a bad area at the time and, seeing as one of its assistant principals was charged with murdering one of its teachers just recently, I'm guessing it probably still is. My classmates and I didn't have a great high school education compared to what we might have gotten in a safer environment. I was bussed into this pretty rough and dangerous school where there were riots, a lack of school resources, and the perils of the neighborhood itself all as distractions from actual learning and education. But the experience motivated me to do better. Do better to be better for myself and for my future. I wanted a different and greater picture of education.

During my high school years, tennis was a healthy outlet for me and many of the other kids in the poor and occasionally violent community. Using that outlet combined with my academics, I started to look toward college. My high school years were very formative, but not in the ways one might think. I was determined to get a degree and have more nurturing and growth-minded experiences for my own children one day. Of course, that's just what I wanted in my mind. I had to actually make it come to fruition, next. In those days, I was a smart kid in a struggling class, but I didn't really excel, per sé. It wasn't an ideal environment for building a successful student path. Success was defined as just getting through it.

When I applied to colleges, I was completely lost. As one of the first people in my family to attend college (and the first to graduate), I applied without letters of recommendation. I didn't know I needed any letters of recommendation. In fact, even more absurdly, I had never even heard of the SAT.

When I was told that I needed to take the SAT to get into college, I signed up for the next test I could find in the area . . . though not at my own school. I walked into the classroom and very quickly felt out of place. Other kids there that day had classes and books and tutors to prepare them. By contrast, they had to provide me with the most basic of tools when I arrived--a pencil--so that I could take the exam. I guess I'd held onto enough knowledge that I managed to do pretty well on the test, though, and—after completing the rest of my requirements to get into college—I was accepted at the University of Minnesota.

When I arrived at orientation, I felt very out of place . . . again. I had hair down the middle of my back; I was tanned (unlike most in the northern university); and—because I was pretty small in stature—my letter jacket came nearly to my knees. I felt physically like a kid next to most of my classmates. I also realized how competitive everyone else on campus was with regard to their athletic abilities.

In a new environment, I realized I would need a new mentality. Thankfully, the competitive attributes that I'd learned in sports came out and I tapped into them to achieve my desire of

> *Thankfully, the competitive attributes that I learned in sports came out, and I really wanted to be smarter, be better, and be at the top of my class.*

becoming smarter, better, and—eventually—at the top of my class. With this new drive, I dove deep into my studying and hard work.

I began succeeding and excelling academically, but I was still competing in tennis in the hopes of becoming a professional player. I was either studying or playing tennis. That was my whole existence in Minnesota. If I wasn't in the books, I would be on the courts in every free moment I had during the day, at night, and on weekends. I was convinced that if I tried harder, worked more, and put in longer hours, I'd be better at the game I loved. But it didn't seem to be happening for me.

There were other athletes who had the right body builds, training, experience, and natural talent to excel in the sport. Some people just have "it" and sometimes "it" is simply genetics, too. There's a reason they are called elite athletes. No matter what I did to change my status, I could not win in the tournaments when it mattered most, and I finally had to face the reality that my dream of being a professional tennis player was not going to happen.

I had to change my vision for my career and everything that I had pictured for my entire life. I only knew that I wanted to do something good and I couldn't think of greater good than being a doctor. Here was the problem: *'How was I going to be a doctor?'*

My whole life, I'd wanted to be a tennis player; I grew up believing I was going to be a tennis player; all my efforts were directed toward being a tennis player. Now I, all of a sudden, wanted to be a doctor? *'Wow,'* I thought. *'This is going to be difficult.'* And indeed, it was.

When I shared my decision with people close to me, many of them shook their heads or rolled their eyes. I didn't have the pedigree to succeed in medical school. I was less qualified for that than a life of tennis! I didn't know anything about medical school. I really didn't even know anything about being a doctor. All I knew was that I couldn't be a tennis player. I'd tried and I accepted this fact. I had to do something with my life and being a doctor sounded like as good an idea as anything. If I couldn't be elite on the tennis courts. I'd be elite in a medical office. Everything I'd poured into tennis now needed to go to this new goal.

Stubbornness for betterment continued to be my constant companion along my path toward a life in medicine. I was accepted to the University of Miami School of Medicine and discovered it to be a cut-throat atmosphere of academic excellence. I felt totally inadequate (again!) and, for the first six weeks, I'd sit as close to the back of the class as possible so that nobody would notice me drowning. I'd jet out as soon as it was over and avoid interacting with any of the other students.

I absorbed all that I could, though, and I worked hard. In time, I adapted and once more found my drive to thrive. I was able to participate in unique opportunities, including an externship in Houston with orthopedics.

These guys were crazy in the best way, especially to a former athlete like me. I dug the adrenaline. We were dealing with current and ex-athletes, broken people and bodies, and—for the first time since starting along the college path—I knew in my heart, finally, *'This is where I belong.'*

This was my kind of medicine and I made the commitment to specialize in orthopedics. I knew that I didn't want to be a general orthopedic doctor; I wanted to be at the top. I wanted to be the best. And I realized that I could marry the worlds I now loved equally: sports and medicine. I knew sports. I knew how athletes thought. I'd lived it (and failed at it). Now, I needed to know medicine . . . and win at it!

With only a small handful of educational opportunities really specializing in sports orthopedics at the time, I was determined to get interviews with the top programs. I spent more than a modest student should to pick up Gucci shoes and a proper suit for my interviews. I wanted to look the part.

Gratefully, I landed a coveted fellowship with Dr. Joseph Torg, a very famous sports medicine legend. He had many achievements including developing *The National Head and Neck Registry for Spinal Cord Injuries in Sports.* Dr. Torg realized that head and neck injuries were caused by spearing and tackling with the crown of the helmet and this is what subsequently caused cervical spinal injuries. This was in the early 1970s. No one had figured this out before him. Dr. Torg was the doctor I chose to learn from, and it was an unbelievable experience.

Dr. Torg had served as team physician for the Philadelphia 76ers, the Philadelphia Flyers, and the Philadelphia Eagles. In addition, his education and research were so well respected that he was chosen as the physician consultant for President Ronald Reagan's Council on Physical Fitness and Sports. I had the opportunity to witness the pace and pressure of this specialized offshoot of orthopedics and sports medicine at the hands of one of its pioneers and I didn't hesitate to realize the honor as I lived it.

I enjoyed the chance to connect with the teams he worked for, and I discovered the close, personal, all-access relationships required of doctors at that level. I worked in a pseudo-assistant team doctor role and I was on call at all times; and I loved it.

My time in Dr. Torg's fellowship led me to more thoroughly understand the world I wanted to make my own. I witnessed the crazy

> *I realized the unbelievably high pressure of caring for some of the world's top athletes.*

pace of daytime work including diagnoses, injection treatments, surgeries, and more. I saw the constant development of research and shared education that one must stay on top of. I realized the unbelievably high pressure of caring for some of the world's top athletes (who are also and often our heroes). I recognized that it was all done without regard for the number of hours required to manage it. I knew that this path would demand a lifetime commitment of staying at the top of my game in order to keep others at the top of theirs. But—to me—it was worth it.

I'm still a huge sports fan and to be able to extend careers, take already phenomenal athletes and make them better, or watch people return to their courts and fields after they thought their careers were over, easily overwhelms the difficult parts of this job with pride and positivity.

I finished my journey to my current role as the Director of the U.S. Center for Sports Medicine. It took me through more education, externships, a residency at Washington University in St. Louis where I met my wife (a surgeon, herself) with whom I would have my children, time spent in a group orthopedic practice before specializing in sports, and numerous opportunities to serve as team doctor to professional sports organizations, Olympic teams, and elite athletes.

It was while I was serving my Orthopedic Surgery Residency at Barnes Hospital/Washington University, in St. Louis, Missouri, that one-time "World's Fastest Man" Ivory Crockett (by then a respected coach) was a patient. I had treated him as a resident, and we had become good friends. We continued our relationship as I moved into my own practice. One day he called and asked me, "Would you do me a favor and look at a young lady's ankle?"

That young lady was Jackie Joyner-Kersee, a track athlete from the struggling community of East St. Louis. She was sister to Olympic Gold Medalist Al Joyner and sister-in-law to Olympic Silver Medalist Florence "Flo-Jo" Griffith-Joyner. Ivory asked if I would meet at the track and, from that time forward,

I have had the joy of working with Jackie. But first I had to earn her trust.

Jackie's one-time coach, Nino Fennoy (who would also become a friend and patient) presented that first step as the biggest challenge in a place like East St. Louis. Nino said, "You have to establish the trust relationship. You do that by enjoying the present opportunity with love and warmth; you meet athletes at their level; you can't live through them; you have to support them; and you care more for the person than for their accomplishments."

Jackie had injured her ankle at the World Championships, and she was home for her Jackie Joyner-Kersee East St. Louis relays. Prior to meeting her and her husband, Bobby Kersee, who would become one of my best friends, I was entrusted with examining her ankle due to the referral from Ivory Crockett. This introduction was one of the most important of my career and I must thank Ivory for this introduction for my friendship with both him and Bobby and Jackie Joyner-Kersee.

Jackie later said, "I was impressed with the way he felt every bone. It wasn't x-rays. He pointed out things I knew, but he didn't. I hadn't told him. It wasn't a guessing game for Doc. I told Bobby that Doc was great, and it wasn't just lip service."

I was detailed when I sat with Jackie and also when I spoke to her coaches. I appreciated the coach's role. I worked meticulously in my lane but didn't forget who was in charge. Sometimes, even team trainers forget that the coach is the coach, but I knew that I had a role to play on the athlete's team and it wasn't "Coach."

Just as Bobby had to trust me, I had to trust him. We would talk for hours. I would watch him explain something about mechanics

> *Doctors should spend more time with elite coaches; coaches are incredible resources.*

of the body and it was really a two-way street. Doctors should spend more time with elite coaches; coaches are incredible resources.

Bobby and I bonded on this journey and bonded over the care of many elite athletes going forward. Bob Kersee and I had a true partnership and this true brotherhood benefitted many athletes. The two of us are like a family still today.

In the words of Nino Fennoy, "Some things are just predestined. Doctor Lehman, me, JJK, Bobby? That's predestination. Doctor Lehman and I have always been on the same page together as part of an athlete support team because we have genuine love and respect for the athletes . . . not the athletic events, but the people. What would I want for my daughter? I wouldn't want anything that would negatively affect her long-term quality of life. With Dr. Lehman, it's never about an event. The health and welfare of the athlete is more important to him."

The most important thing that this unique team shared was an understanding that the health and welfare of the athlete was paramount. This was not about a moment in time; this was about a lifetime. This authentic approach of placing the athlete's lifetime needs first needs to permeate the athlete, the athlete's family, the doctor, and the coach. This is the core foundation of a healthy athlete-care relationship.

◆◆◆◆◆◆

"J, trust me," I told her. "It's gonna be okay."

Getting back to 1996.

It did take all of us to get Jackie ready, but—to be clear—that week was all her. Her mind was as strong as her body. We worked on her nonstop while the rest of the Olympics went on.

The stadium was tense during the event. Jackie was stone-faced as she paced anxiously before her first jump. Her leg was taped, and her initial jumps were very difficult for her. On her last jump, with ultimate anticipation from the crowd, Jackie pulled off a jump of seven meters[1].

---

[1]Hart, Rodney (Author), and Eric Draper (Photographer). "Jackie-Joyner Kersee to Be in Quincy for Bridge The Gap To Health in May, Agility Camp in June." Harold-Whig, The Harold-Whig, 24 Mar. 2010.

Jackie's jump was good enough to put her on the podium and it may have been one of her career's biggest accomplishments. In her typical complete professionalism, Jackie waved to the crowd, a proud Olympian who had literally leapt over competitors to earn a spot on the podiums for her final time. It was an immeasurable honor to be a part of such an incredible part of sports history.

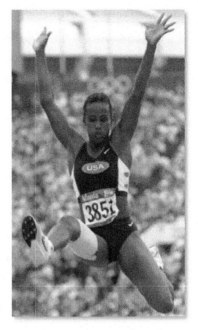

Photo: "Jackie Joyner-Kersee performs during the 1996 Olympic Games in Atlanta. (AP Photo)."
www.whig.com/article/20100324/ARTICLE/303249982. Accessed 20 Jul. 2020.

◆◆◆◆◆◆

Jackie's comeback and my relationship with the Kersees matter because they are central to my philosophy and approach to orthopedics and sports medicine. Being in Jackie's life as her doctor has been about more than belonging to a championship team. Jackie's and Bobby's lessons have carried through my lifelong practice.

- They have helped to shape my understanding of athletic preparation, development, and maintenance.
- They have introduced me to the concept of teamwork, not just on the fields and courts of play, but in the lives and support networks of athletes.
- They have helped me recognize the types of expectations that we can set (and who should set them) at the different stages of an athlete's career.
- They have shown me—in action—the roles of minds, hearts, and emotions in sports performance.
- I have learned about the power of general health and nutrition disciplines, as well as how to overcome injury and illness from stress and trauma.
- They have taught me above all that—in order to be an elite sports medicine physician—I have to stay ahead of the curve, be inventive, and be on the cutting edge of my field (which is exactly what we expect of our athletes).

The Formula

What I've noticed over the course of my career bears passing on to ensure the health, safety, and both the career- and life-longevities of our athletes. Most of what I've witnessed, learned, and practiced leads me to understand the sentinel underlying component of elite athletics: Olympic athletes and world-class athletes are born; they cannot be cultivated. If you have the basic underlying talent, success comes by utilizing a cooperative team, and every component of an athlete's team must be present for that athlete to succeed.

The perception and direction of sports has gone awry at every level. Back in the early glory days of professional sports in the 1960s, athletes had jobs in their off seasons. Working in their sport was their honor; not their primary livelihood. The whole financial undertone has changed sports and the trickle-down effect it has had on all aspects of our athlete management has been terrible.

We need to play to our kids' strengths. If your kid loves to swim and that's the strength, let him swim. Who cares if there's no money or scholarships in it? Who cares if it doesn't have a following or a career field? What I've seen happen instead is that the fame and fortune elements of athletics have ushered in mystique and adoration for the lifestyles we associate with professional sports. Those lifestyles have become the goals rather than the sports that could get them there.

- Kids see professional athletes and they are entertained.
- Parents see the glamorous lives and want them for their kids.
- Coaches see heroes and want to be credited with creating them.
- Doctors see champions and let kids play who shouldn't.

The pop and pizzazz of pro sports have taken away from fun, safe, enjoyable fitness. People around young athletes put undue pressure on them to build careers in fields that have a limited lifespan, very little "shelf-space," and can potentially result in long-term physical and emotional damage. It's important to understand that the careers of most professional athletes are very short, injury is a probability (not just a possibility), and the emotional impacts can be life-altering.

I've seen parents try to turn their sons and daughters into seekers of pots of gold and lights of glory. This can lead their children to depression and feelings of failure. What's worse is that, in the

> *In the pushing, pressuring, and power-grabbing, we are destroying their bodies (and sometimes minds), making it even less likely that they will make it in the long run.*

pushing, pressuring, and power-grabbing, we are destroying their bodies (and sometimes minds), making it even less likely that they will make it in the long run (even if that was the athlete's initial desire, and not just the wish of the parents).

If your kid isn't going to be a professional, how can you still encourage them to do sports for all the good that they can get from that participation?

MY MISSIONS FOR THIS BOOK ARE:

- *One—it teaches us to work toward building an athlete to have his or her greatest potential for success in sports.*
- *Two—it offers a guide toward building a successful member of society, having utilized the immense positives of mental and physical training toward a goal.*
- *Three—it maximizes success in life.*

Sports, approached with the methods discussed in this book, allow people to be leaders; they allow people to have mental and physical direction; and they teach us the ability to succeed. If one can learn the lessons of succeeding in athletics, one can succeed in life and break through the glass ceilings we all face.

There are a lot of great reasons for being involved in sports and going pro shouldn't be the only one. It can be a goal and hope, but there must be a greater purpose for sports involvement because professional endeavors are probably the least likely of outcomes to occur.

Even if an athlete doesn't go pro, there are still many very important things to be gained from sports: discipline, hard work, learning how to bust through when you've got nothing left to give, interpersonal skills, and more. These are life experiences, not just resumé experiences, and we should let our young people have them!

What you will learn in the following pages comes from more than 35 years of medical experience in treating some of the world's greatest athletes. I've been able to see what has worked and what has not worked; and I have been able to see total success and total failure. Hopefully, these lessons will help to guide you in the upbringing of your children athletes and building a healthy relationship that is enduring.

The formula to R.A.I.S.E. an athlete includes:

R.EALISTIC EXPECTATIONS –

What is the course of your athlete's future in his or her sport and how can you best prepare him or her for success along that path?

A.VOID DANGERS AND PITFALLS –

Avoid the dangers of unhealthy habits, drug abuse, and abnormal relationships. We need to avoid the dark side of sports.

I.NJURY AND ILLNESS MANAGEMENT

Discover the common and lesser-known injuries and illnesses athletes face in their sports, as well as how to heal from them.

S.EGUE TO LIFE AFTER SPORTS

Build an understanding of the longevity of a sports career (amateur, academic, or professional) and ensure your athlete has the skills to have a successful life off and after the fields and courts of play.

E.NJOY THE GAME

Learn to appreciate all of the good that comes from sports and athletic endeavors beyond trophies and treasures.

R.ealistic Expectations

The Numbers

et's get concrete. The unfortunate reality is that a kid is more likely to be born with an extra digit—the odds are 1 in 500—than they are to become a professional athlete. Here are the numbers for some top sports, ones organized by high-paying leagues and organizations.[2] Keep in mind, these figures represent the highest probability of becoming a professional athlete, along the most traditional course: high school to college to professional league.

FOOTBALL
- 1 in 40 high school players will play football in college (2.5%)
- 1 in 325 college players will play in the NFL (0.3%)
- 3 out of every 40,000 players go professional on the traditional route (.0075%)

---

[2] Julian Sonny, "The Statistical Breakdown of Becoming a Professional Athlete Will Make You Keep Your Day Job," Elite Daily, Bustle Digital Group, Feb. 26, 2014, https://www.elitedaily.com/sports/odds-going-pro-sports-will-make-rethink-day-job.

MEN'S BASKETBALL

- 1 in 17 high school players will play basketball in college (5.8%)
- 1 in 525 college players will play in the NBA (0.1%)
- 29 out of every 500,000 players go professional on the traditional route (.0058%)

WOMEN'S BASKETBALL

- 1 in 16 high school players will play basketball in college (6.3%)
- 1 in 766 college players will play in the WNBA (0.1%)
- 63 out of every Million players go professional on the traditional route (.0063%)

MEN'S BASEBALL

- 1 in 9 high school players will play baseball in college (11%)
- 1 in 44 college players will play baseball in the MLB (2.3%)
- 253 out of every 100,000 players go professional on the traditional route (.253%)

WOMEN'S SOFTBALL

- 1 in 13 high school players will play softball in college (7.7%)

- 1 in 1,484 college players will play softball in the NPF (0.06%)
- 231 out of every 5 Million players go professional on the traditional route (.0046%)

MEN'S SOCCER

- 1 in 9 high school players will play soccer in college (9.1%)
- 1 in 447 college players will play soccer in the MLS (0.2%)
- 91 out of every 500,000 players go professional on the traditional route (.0182%)

WOMEN'S SOCCER

- 1 in 10 high school players will play soccer in college (10%)
- 1 in 986 college players will play soccer in the NWSL (0.1%)
- 1 out of every 10,000 players go professional on the traditional route (.01%)

MEN'S HOCKEY

- 1 in 9 high school players will play hockey in college (11%)
- 1 in 20 college players will play hockey in the NHL (5%)
- 11 out of every 2,000 players go professional on the traditional route (.55%)

WOMEN'S HOCKEY

- These statistics are still somewhat soft as the WNHL is a relatively new league, but there are only six teams in the full league. They choose from players across the world and only 1 in 4 (25%) of U.S. high school players go on to play in college. Preliminary statistics point to a less than 5% likelihood of becoming professional in this sport.

These statistics were all pre-COVID and we have yet to see what the long-term fallout that the professional sports' stoppages will have on recruiting, attrition, and success probabilities, but—if they reflect the rest of the world—things may become even tighter. Additionally, the probability of "making it" is only one of the statistics that play into the success of a professional athlete.

◆ ◆ ◆ ◆ ◆ ◆

If one does manage to "make it" in the big leagues, there's still the issue of managing money. I've seen hundreds of athletes live out exceptional professional careers, only to wind up broke. That's the reality of professional sports: getting in is hard, staying long is unlikely, and getting out is no guarantee that you're set for life.

Sports Illustrated estimated that 78 percent of NFL players are bankrupt or financially stressed within two years of retirement. The NBA doesn't fare much better: 60 percent are penniless within five years of leaving the sport.[3] *(2017)*

There are a number of reasons for these unfortunate statistics. For many athletes, their professional salary must support an entire extended family. That, of course, is fine and noble, until the group relying on the athlete expands to not-so-close family, friends, and community members who feel entitled to a slice of the success. While it's very generous and well-intended for young, newly wealthy athletes to buy expensive gifts for his or her friends, it's not the prudent financial decision. Rather than ooh and aah over celebrity athletes living a high-rolling lifestyle—which never lasts—we should coach our athletes to set aside a percentage of their earnings each year, so that they're not forced to struggle in their later years, when their royalties have dwindled and their bodies are used up from professional wear and tear in their younger years.

Of course, it's not just family, friends, and fans who are the problem. From an early age, many talented athletes are saddled with a bloated staff of agents, assistants, administrators, lawyers, insurance and tax

---

[3] Brooks, Rodney. "Why Do so Many Pros Go Broke?" The Undefeated, The Undefeated, 28 Mar. 2017, theundefeated.com/features/why-do-so-many-pros-go-broke/.

preparers, advisors and other professional encourage members all drawn to the athlete's power and financial largess. Most of these individuals mean well and are themselves running legitimate ventures, but in aggregate, they drain the athlete's resources quickly. Athletes should consider retaining only the most necessary support and advisors, who have the individual's best interest at heart and who respect and honor his or her long-term financial plan. The support team kept should be the one that will help the athlete achieve his or her professional goals during and after a sports career.

Put simply, athletes need to learn to live by the same money-management skills expected of any working adult. If an athlete has a shot at the big time and wants to pursue it, adopting a realistic and informed stance on "making it" is not only smart—it's necessary.

◆◆◆◆◆◆

Let's take some time to dig into the players on the team who are non-negotiable—the family, the coach, and the medical staff—because even Jackie Joyner-Kersee didn't get become a track legend on her own.

In line with realistic expectations, there are a few things to keep in mind: one—great athletes are born;

two—what athletes choose to do with their talent, their team, their family, their mental and physical guidance, and their determination collectively decides their success; and three—although the odds are low, many athletes (in raw numbers, not percentages) will get scholarships and some not rare numbers of athletes will play professional sports. Furthermore, regardless of whether an athlete intends to have a professional career in sports, an education is a valuable benefit that can be supported by sports and is in itself a definition of success.

A young athlete with potential to be a professional will propel much further with encouragement, rather than pressure. Attention must be paid toward building the complete dynamics of both the athlete and a productive member of society.

Athletes can both participate in sports and develop other interests and passions. Family can promote the professional athletic path and help to develop a well-rounded citizen. Coaches can train for an event but must also serve as teachers who need to teach about the complexities of life. Doctors can heal an athlete for a game or season, but, much more importantly, should work to maintain a lifelong health outlook for the patient and be protective of the athlete's life post-athletic career.

The Family

The second member of an athlete's team, after the athlete himself or herself, is family. The athlete's family is typically comprised of parents or guardians, especially when the athlete is young and in need of others to inform, guide toward, or make important decisions. For some athletes, adult mentors and leaders fill that familial role on the athlete's team. The singular most important role of parents and guardians is to parent! They must raise that human before trying to build that athlete.

> *"During the time I was coming up through school, girls in sports were frowned upon. My mom didn't really know what I did athletically,"* Jackie confessed.

> *"Mom wanted me to get an education and a job. If an activity interfered with homework or cleaning my room, it was secondary. But my dad told me it was good for me. There had to be a balance to keep my priorities in order. Go on the weekends to practices and keep up my schooling and chores during the week. My parents couldn't*

> *always attend my practices, either. They were young and dad and mom were teenagers trying to raise a family."*

I know it sounds simple, but I've so often seen mothers and fathers who are working more in the role of talent management than in parenthood. They are the driving force behind the

> *The job of an athlete's parent is not to establish the foundation for a sports career; it is to establish the foundation for a productive and caring member of society.*

sport participant (which, if you recall, is the role of the athlete). They are pursuing scholarships and professionalism on behalf of their sons or daughters who may or may not want them. This is not to say they shouldn't help an athlete with that desire; but the desire, itself, should come from the child. Parents are sometimes asking about their athletes' next steps in a potential athletic career in adulthood while their sons and daughters are more concerned about asking someone out on a date the next week. The job of an athlete's parent is not to establish the foundation for a sports career; it is to establish the foundation for a productive and caring member of society, and this is inclusive of supporting their child's respective sport.

The family should be working toward building respectable values in the athlete's life, not just athletic success. The parents' priorities should be to love their child first, and—only in a secondary goal—support his or her sports accomplishments. By the time athletes are in college, they should be prepared to have responsibility for themselves and that responsibility is learned through watching and experiencing the leadership of family in their own lives.

Coach Jay Harrington, Junior College Baseketball Coach, states that he has uncomfortable conversations with parents every single day because that's his job. Being what—on its surface—seems like the bad guy. In reality, he's being a protector. Sometimes a dad or mom is willing to go along with an eager kid who is injured and should be pulled, for instance. They may even be proud that their son or daughter is willing to suck it up, get out there, and push through the pain.

I, as an orthopedic surgeon, often feel as Coach Harrington—that I have to act as a protector. I have to protect the athlete from long-term damage and ensure that they have a very healthy life after sports.

Kids will only put up with so much and, after a while, enough is enough: enough pain, enough pressure, and enough of the sport, entirely. I'll change the environment when I can, change the pressure. I've seen too many kids, high-level athletes, whose families put everything into their child becoming a pro. At times, this is not realistic.

It's true that the athlete is the first member of the athlete's team, but the family is actually the leading member of the team. Taking that lead role on the team is the most important task for parents and family. In order to accomplish leadership successfully, the parent(s) must understand the roles of each person on the team and ensure nobody is stepping on anybody else's toes. Make sure the coach isn't circumventing recommendations from a doctor and have the parents quarterback the functions of each member of the athlete's team: athlete, coaches, and doctors.

In the case when a parent is also a coach, which is more likely to occur at the youngest ages rather than further along in an athlete's career, the approach is simple. In practice and games, that parent is a coach. At all other times, that parent is family. Don't parent on the field or coach around the dinner table. Hopefully, the parents in this unique position have the ability to recognize the full teams around every one of their athletes.

It's also important that parents build relationships with the other team members ensuring they have shared goals. In this endeavor, it falls to family to keep open communications between all members of the team. Particularly if the medical team does not have a relationship with the coaching staff, it is the responsibility of the parents to relay important information about the athlete's physical needs. The leadership-level of involvement from the family can be hard to maintain, but—when executed with honesty and frequent open communication—it both respects the important roles of others and honors the primary role parents have for the athlete: to parent the child with love.

◆◆◆◆◆◆

PEER PRESSURE

Peer pressure—the influence a kid or young adult feels from their peers to behave a certain way—is nothing new, but in today's world, with the prevalence of social media, it's an important problem to discuss. With considered action and involvement, parents and family (and coaches as well) can help mitigate the spread and negative effects of peer pressure.

To be clear, peer pressure isn't always bad. When it drives an athlete to train harder—he doesn't want to let his teammates down, or she dives for that drop shot because her school is counting on her—it can be a helpful, positive force. If it's pushing an athlete toward drugs, steroids, unrealistic body images, or other harmful activities, like bullying or hazing, that's when it becomes a problem.

Problematic peer pressure often rears its head in high school, when teenage athletes are starting to carve out their own identities. The best thing a parent can do to avoid this kind of peer pressure is talk regularly to their kids and build up their self-esteem and self-compassion. Parents should be stable, trusting, and non-judgmental. I realize it can sound trite, but frequent touch-ins from parents can help teenagers think independently from those around them, and make choices about what they think is right, and not what others think is acceptable or cool. This kind of independent thinking also helps teenagers develop a leadership mentality, which is one of the great benefits of playing sports in the first place.

Technology is simply another avenue by which negative social pressures reach our kids. Anyone can go online and post a bunch of harmful messages which they would never articulate in person. The recipient of those nasty messages, though, feels just as bad as if they'd heard them face-to-face. Meanwhile, the sender of the messages doesn't get the instant negative feedback of seeing the other person hurt. The reality of putting unfeeling technology between words written and words read creates a vicious cycle based in a lack of human empathy and an increase of human callousness. Such behaviors undercut the self-esteem and confidence a family tries to instill in young athletes. Social media has the positive of being able to connect people in different countries, but it can drive a wedge between teammates standing right next to each other.

So how can parents and families help? Talk to your young athlete. Let them know you understand that they're dealing with both the real world and the digital one. Share your own experiences in navigating the differences between interacting with human beings and posting things on social media. Encourage them to share with you.

An unfortunate reality of the pandemic is that much of the country and world was sent online and told that it was the same as being in person. It has been a functional reality, but it cannot be a long-term one. While we all had to accept certain things in the name of public health, we will need to remind our young—as in-person activities and gatherings come back into play—that interpersonal connections are more valuable than internet connections. Validate their desire to participate in the current digital environment, while also letting them know that there is no substitute for real-life interactions . . . something they should feel grateful for getting back to very soon.

Giving a young athlete the tools to balance their digital and real-world lives at home will make it more likely that they'll have success doing the same at school and in their sports.

The Guide

Over the years, dozens of parents have asked me for a succinct guide to managing their athletic sons and daughters. I'm not a parenting expert—just ask my three kids—but having treated thousands of kids of all ages, below is just such a guide: a way for parents to think about the different stages of their young athletes' lives.

AGES 5 TO 8

Developmental Description
At this early stage, most children are naturally upbeat. They don't fatigue easily and will wear their emotions on their sleeves. Young kids are watchers and copiers—they will do as you do, and not as you say.

How to Incorporate Sports
- Ask your kid what they're interested in and build their athletic activities around those interests.

- Make suggestions where you see gifts or talent but allow the child to make his own choices.
- Offer all kinds of activities, not just sports.
- Try to engage your child in a mix of individual and team activities.
- Coaches should focus on fitness, fun, and basic skills.

What Parents Can Do

- Look out for bullying and opportunities to teach kids self-advocacy.
- Talk to your kids! They love to tell you about themselves at this age, so listen. Don't shy away from heavy subjects; just discuss them at levels your child can understand.
- If your kid brings up a sports hero, comment on your admiration that she or he doesn't use drugs, and on their work ethic, rather than just their athletic achievements.
- Do things with your kid other than sports activities: read, walk, and get involved in your community. Let them know they matter regardless of athletic achievements.
- In sports, reward participation and effort, not results: *'You ran so hard out there!' 'You really watched that ball!' 'You looked like you were having fun!'*

- As far as nutrition, the biggest thing for little kids is carb control. Introduce high protein breakfasts, mild to moderate carbs, and vegetables that kids will learn to like.

Do This

- Set patterns and routines. Patterns become habits, and habits make a difference in long-term success. Establish schedules with activities and boundaries; kids need certainty and consistency. Repetition is great at this stage and more important than variety.

AGES 9 TO 12

Developmental Description

This is a highly transitional phase. Some kids start to mature and, by age 12, are grown; others may remain biologically and psychologically young. Males and females will have different issues and will require different parenting strategies. Friendships begin to play a larger role. Outside relationships will develop; parents begin to share influence over their child's life with others. Technology becomes a part of a child's life at this stage (if not before) at least through schooling and perhaps even at a social level; parents need a plan for managing screen time.

How to Incorporate Sports

- Kids should learn foundational skills in these years.

- Allow children to try different sports. Variety is healthy at this stage; children should still not specialize in a single sport.

- Give kids off-seasons; they shouldn't have organized sports year-round. They should learn that sports can be fun without being a competition.

- Teach your kids about engaging with sports outside of play. Show them how to be a fan. Point out the other people involved in the game (referees, coaches, doctors, statisticians, reporters, etc.). Let kids see sports from many sides so they don't see winning as the only form of success.

- Encourage sports for recreation and socialization; family outings and gatherings of friends are great for fitness and emotional well-being.

What Parents Can Do

- Talk to your kids about differences and changes in biology.

- For girls, who will typically mature toward the start of this phase, discuss nutrition. Emphasize health and strength rather than weight and body shape. Make sure they understand the biology of their feelings and have frank conversations about depression, regression, isolation, and self-image.

- For boys, who will typically mature toward the end of this phase, explain the normalcy of emotional changes and how to channel feelings positively. Help them understand anger, emotional swings, aggressive tendencies brought about by hormones, and frustration, and provide positive outlets for those feelings.

- Statistically speaking, though not exclusively, girls will tend more toward depression and anxiety, whereas boys will tend more toward anger. Both extremes can result in psychologically unhealthy behaviors ranging from anxiety, to addictions, to self-harm, to violence. Talk openly with them; let them know they shouldn't be ashamed and to come to you about these important issues before their feelings become negative actions.

- Moderate your child's screen time and social media activity. Set guidelines early and be familiar with their digital environments. You're training your child to protect their own privacy as they get older.

- Encourage friendships, but reserve space for family time in which you celebrate and demonstrate the values you wish to instill.

- Build habits that prioritize fitness, nature, nutrition, and proper sleep. You're still in charge (though it may not feel like it).

- Maintain a normal eating schedule with regular meals (that don't continue past 10 o'clock at night) but allow for flexibility. (Your kid shouldn't feel bad about the occasional fast-food meal with friends or snacking late at a sleepover.)

- Remember: your kid is still watching you. If you smoke, your child is 29[4] percent more likely to smoke, as well. Your negative choices in general are more likely to become your child's actions than you wish to believe.

model

AGES 13 TO 15

Developmental Description

Welcome to the toughest phase of parenthood. There's a lot going on at this age. There will be bad days for both you and your child. Look for longer patterns of sadness, depression, and isolation in your child. Kids start going out in the world at this stage: it's the parents' job to maintain and nurture their relationship with their children.

---

[4] "Study: Teens' Smoking Influenced by Older Siblings, Parents' Lifelong Smoking Habits." *Purdue University*, www.purdue.edu/newsroom/releases/2013/Q3/study-teens-smoking-influenced-by-older-siblings,-parents-lifelong-smoking-habits.html.

How to Incorporate Sports

- Let your kids specialize in a chosen sport, but don't have them spend the full year doing it. Off-seasons and variety are healthy.

- Emphasize (positive) competitiveness, fitness, and strength. Be mindful of negative obsessions over winning.

- Connect through sports by going to live or one-on-one events with your child.

What Parents Can Do

- Be in their lives. You should be the go-to when they struggle in sports and in life.

- Communication is harder. It's your job to go behind "Yes," "No," "Okay," and "Fine," in conversations.

- Ask open-ended questions that encourage the child to elaborate. Once they start sharing details, they'll look forward to sharing with you more often because you'll have the background. Communication can develop its own snowball effect.

- Nutrition is harder to control because fewer foods are consumed at home. Provide what you can, encourage them to make good choices, and check in with them regularly.

- Keep healthy, convenient snacks in the house. If they can grab it on the go, they're more likely to eat it.

- Don't assume your child understands what a carb, a protein, or a fat is. Educate them. Talk to them about "fake" health foods and supplements.

- Learn about metabolism together. Kids, especially high-performing athletes, need to eat an appropriate amount of nutritionally valuable food every day. They also need to hydrate and maintain electrolytes. Teach them to nourish for strength and health so that they value this more than eating (or not eating) for appearance.

- Encourage kindness and in-person connection between your child and their friends. In these years, teens often grapple with self-centeredness, groupthink, and a need to prove oneself. Help them to develop outward thinking.

AGES 16 TO 18

Developmental Description

Separation is normal at this stage. Your kid is honing a self-image; you have less control over their decisions. This is a good time to begin building a friendship with your child and take a supporting role in their life.

How to Incorporate Sports

- If your child plays sports, set realistic expectations in casual conversation. Encourage their continued participation, but don't pressure them. Make sure they understand that athletics are not the only path to success.

- Talk to your child about practice, games, and events. Regularly ask them how they feel, both physically and emotionally.

- Ask open-ended questions and make space for them to ask questions in return.

- Be the cheerleader; not the coach.

What Parents Can Do

- Continue to be an example of good nutrition, fitness for the sake of health and strength.

- Demonstrate and encourage proper sleep.

- Your best contribution at this stage is not as a teacher, but as a supporter and model of proper habits.

- Keep open communications with the rest of your child's athletic team—coaches and trainers, medical professionals, and educators.

- If your kid doesn't want to play sports anymore—because they don't enjoy it, or they've lost their sense of self-worth outside of athletics—let them leave. Offer love so your child doesn't feel that your acceptance was predicated on their performance as an athlete. Ask questions, without guiding your kid toward a particular answer. Encourage your kid to have conversations with teachers and coaches so that they are making a logically and emotionally informed decision. You are not the only adult in their life and this talk is sometimes easier with a non-parent.

GROWN COLLEGIATE ATHLETES

Developmental Description
Now, you're truly in the role of supporter. Be friends and confidantes to your kids and respect them as adult individuals. Get to know their roommates, teammates, coaches, teachers, and friends. And always keep talking to them!

How to Incorporate Sports
- If your kid child gives up a college sport, there may be emotional struggles. Listen, be attuned, and—if necessary, seek professional help (for which there is no stigma).

- Most athletes will know if they aren't making it to the next level—and that's okay! No college student should feel that he or she failed because they didn't "go pro."

- If your kid wants to be involved in sports but won't make it in the pros, talk with them about other careers, possibly around sports, while encouraging them to enjoy their sport for what it provides outside of a career path.

- If your kid is done with sports, help them find joy in exercise, fitness, and the activities that make them happy.

What Parents Can Do

- Love your kids. Lay the groundwork for a successful future regardless of sports

- Look at the big picture. Your behavior has a profound impact on your child's life, and your relationship with them.

◆◆◆◆◆◆

Regardless of the age of an athlete, an important job of parents is building the rest of the team: identify coaches and medical staff that will help their young athlete. All parties are responsible for communication and cooperation, but as the nucleus of the support team, it's the family's job to lead the charge.

The Coaches

In the 1970s and '80s, USA Gymnastics trained its young, female athletes with Cold War efficiency. Coaches pushed, drove, and yelled, striving to sculpt bodies that would perfectly execute on beam, bars, and vault.

In 1982, at the age of fourteen, rising gymnastic star Mary Lou Retton left high school to train under Romanian powerhouses Béla and Márta Károlyi at their ranch in Houston. Soon, thousands of other Olympic hopefuls followed. For decades, USA Gymnastics sent its top performers to Bela and Márta. If you were serious about gymnastics, you went to the ranch.

Retton never spoke out against the Károlyis, but it's now common knowledge that their "ranch" was the site of systemic verbal, emotional, and occasionally physical abuse. Retton herself was once told to sleep off a knee injury which later required emergency surgery—the first of nearly twenty such operations she would eventually require. The ranch, and USA gymnastics more broadly, were toxic environments. Coaches burned through forty or fifty girls in the hopes of finding one or two national heroes. The consequences, which have been widely documented, speak for themselves—systems like this do irreparable and—in some cases—lifelong damage to our young athletes.

Patrick Hulliung, a world-class gymnastics coach (and long-time friend), calls it like it is: "The culture was 'win at all costs.'" Hulliung is emphatic that USA Gymnastics' version of winning—identifying and training gold medal winners—was not worth the cost. "USA Gymnastics separated families. It pushed girls until all of them—including the champions—hated the sport. It broke these girls' bodies before they were even thirty. Is that winning?"

USA Gymnastics may be an extreme example, but the win-at-all-costs mentality existed (and still exists) throughout all sports, and this model of coaching is a broken one. We have to find a way for coaches to inspire and motivate their athletes without harming and breaking them.

The good news is that it's possible: coaches like Patrick Hulliung, Nino Fennoy, Bobby Kersee, and Jay Harrington—men's basketball coach at Southwestern Illinois College—prove this out. I asked these gentlemen what coaches need to do to create a new, positively charged, sustainable model of raising and training our young athletes. Here's some of the advice direct from these best-of-the-best leaders.

TREAT ATHLETES LIKE HUMAN BEINGS

Patrick Hulliung has coached some of the world's most elite gymnasts, including those competing at the highest levels. To him, none of that matters unless he's coaching the right way. "The top is going to be the top, no matter what," he says. "But don't dispose of the others along the way. Build human beings and build character."

As a coach, Hulliung emphasizes health, fitness, and positive affirmation. For him, it's more important for his athletes to learn things like time management, respect, and teamwork, than it is for them to bring home medals.

Nino Fennoy, Jackie's track coach before Bobby, thinks of things the same way. When Jackie wanted to compete in Women's Nationals and Worlds at the age of just fourteen, Fennoy wouldn't let her. "If it's meant to be," he told her, "it will be. If it's meant to be, you'll make the national team as a senior." Then, when Jackie graduated high school, instead of trying to hold onto her as an athlete, he told her, "I've taught you all I can. Now you have to grow and learn from someone else."

Looking back on her relationship with Coach Fennoy, Jackie understands that he prioritized her long-term health over short-term performance, and her development as an adult over his own desire to continue coaching her. To her, it's made all the difference in the world and she felt cared for as a human being, much like Hulliung's gymnasts felt for him.

COACH EACH ATHLETE DIFFERENTLY

It doesn't matter if it's Allyson Felix, Gail Devers, or Jackie. Bobby is the best of the best—his Olympians have brought home more than forty medals—not because he has a magic, one-size-fits-all approach, but because he builds a unique plan around each athlete. He's not running a gymnastics factory, like they were at the Károlyi ranch. His method is that he doesn't have one. "Some coaches and trainers will do A, B, and C every time," he says. "But sometimes what's needed is D or E. You gotta work through and figure out what's right for each person."

Bobby meets with his athletes and their families. He maps out a plan, including what will happen a week, a month, and a year out. He works out what obstacles an athlete might face and what could go wrong. He figures out how to get around those obstacles, which won't be the same for every athlete.

This requires an intense and intimate understanding of the individual—and that's where Bobby shines.

PREPARE ATHLETES FOR LIFE OFF THE COURT

For Jay Harrington, coaching is much more than what happens on the court: it's what happens in his athletes' lives. He's much more interested in raising student athletes than he is in creating scoring machines.

"I teach my players how to be respectful. I guide them on how to dress and carry themselves. I teach discipline and loyalty."

Harrington is tough when he needs to be, but love underpins all of his actions. He knows that what he says and does will stay with his athletes long after they've graduated from college.

"Not all of your athletes will play for money. You have to get them ready for life after sports."

◆◆◆◆◆◆

If coaches can treat their athletes like the unique human beings they are, and understand that young people need to be set up for long-term success in life, then we can start moving away from the systemically abusive systems of the 1970s, '80s, (and beyond), and create a new culture that raises up more than athletes in all sports; it raises up human beings.

BULLYING AND VIOLENCE

As a final note in this coaching section, I want to take a moment to address bullying. While families and medical professionals may see the aftermath of bullying, coaches are on the front lines of where it often occurs and, therefore, in the driver's seat to help prevent it.

Bullying is physical or psychological aggression of one person against another, usually perpetrated against individuals or groups who don't meet some status quo or expected norm. It can be triggered by any number of things—size, appearance, physical ability, or background—and it is particularly rampant among adolescents. It's critical that we dismantle bullying in our sports.

People who bully usually do so because they are taught bigotries which need to be untaught or because they feel threatened. Take as an example a seventeen-year-old captain of the high school tennis team who feels anxious or challenged by an upstart freshman. The insecurities felt by the captain could lead to aggressions against the freshman.

Let's encourage our players to be leaders, to welcome their younger teammates with enthusiasm. Let's make it known that we accept all shapes, sizes,

> *Let's make it known that we accept all shapes, sizes, genders, races, backgrounds, and walks of life.*

genders, races, backgrounds, and walks of life. Coaches are the perfect person for this role; they can lead by example, showing our younger athletes how we should treat one another. They unteach improper stereotypes and model positivity and acceptance.

When the older athletes see this, they will demonstrate it as the established team behavior and culture. Older players' roles as mentors can serve the dual purpose of addressing their insecurities by providing leadership opportunities and also preventing the bullying of new team members.

Now, on violence. Some sports, like football, rugby, lacrosse, and hockey, have some violence by nature. The plays are aggressive and physical. Other activities, like tennis or swimming, generally aren't violent. Like bullying, violence and aggression in competition can result in physical and psychological harm that extends well beyond the field.

In 2006, medical researchers studying young, college-aged men, released a paper showing a link between participation in aggressive high school sports—like football, lacrosse, and hockey—and physical, psychological, and even sexual aggression toward romantic partners.[5] These men were more likely to injure their romantic partners, were more accepting of violence, and held more sexist and hostile attitudes towards women and homosexuality. In other words, if you're violent on the field, there is a higher likelihood of being violent off the field. Because we're trying to raise responsible, societally conscious adults, that's not a good thing.

◆◆◆◆◆◆

Tony Twist, NHL legend and one-time enforcer for the St. Louis Blues hockey team, knows about violence in sports firsthand. In his ten years as a pro hockey player, he suffered more concussions than he can count. It was his role to start, and often end, fights on the ice. Watching old YouTube videos of him, you're surprised that he never killed anybody. It's hard to see. Today, when you shake his hand, accompanied by gentleness and what seems an uncharacteristically warm smile, it's like gripping a gnarled tree branch.

---

[5] Forbes GB, Adams-Curtis LE, Pakalka AH, White KB. Dating aggression, sexual coercion, and aggression-supporting attitudes among college men as a function of participation in aggressive high school sports. Violence Against Women. 2006;12(5):441-455. doi:10.1177/1077801206288126

Every single day that I wake up," Tony Twist says, "I'm still earning that paycheck from 20 years ago. I don't think that 17-year-old hockey player knew that would be the case."

Twist believes that kids in general tend toward aggression in sports. Young hockey players, for instance, are cheered and rewarded for fighting. There is honor in being put into the penalty box. We, the spectators, fans, families, and coaches, are reinforcing negative behavior during games and it's hard for young athletes to turn off the desire for that response outside of their sports. We need to retrain our athletes' brains and stop rewarding them for beating the crap out of each other.

Twist is long retired from the NHL. Today, he's a parent and coach working to create safer, more well-rounded athletic environments than the ones in which he grew up. He believes that coaches can play an impactful role in noticing, and putting an end to, unnecessary bullying and violence with a few simple steps.

- Reward successful non-violence. *'Hey guys, how about that speed Jack had out there today!'*
- Verbally recognize good plays, not just hard hits. Instead of, *'Good job taking out that other player,'* try, *'The way you handled that situation was incredible!'*

- Force players to build one another up. *'Joe, why don't you work with Will on his footwork?'*

- Ask about players' lives outside the arena. *'Jack, how's your older brother doing? I heard he's engaged.'*

- Recognize kids for all achievements, not just athletic ones. *'How about a high five for Hank on his ACT score.'*

◆◆◆◆◆◆

The bottom line regarding violence and bullying in sports is that we can't remove the physical aspects of some of our kids' activities. We are obligated, however, to change the way we coach our players so that aggressive actions don't find their ways into the other aspects of an athlete's life.

Combined with a loving human approach to every athlete, this model for coaching will build better people. As a positive side effect, better people make better athletes and better teams.

A.voiding Dangers and Pitfalls

The Medical Staff

Now that we've taken a look at the athlete, the family, and the coach, it's time to turn our attention to the fourth and final member of our athletic team and the one that I know best: the medical staff.

In my private medical practice—the U.S. Center for Sports Medicine in St. Louis—we're proud to have a variety of expertise. My partner is Dr. Steven Stahle, a sports medicine-trained general practitioner. We employ a host of nurses, technicians, and administrators, all willing to go the extra mile for our patients. Across the hall is Patrick Huck, a physical therapist experienced in helping athletes recover fully and quickly. (Incidentally, my wife, Dr. Michele Koo, a nationally recognized, board-certified plastic surgeon, manages her own private practice and skincare business in the same building). If we don't know exactly how to treat an athlete, mentally and physically, we know the people who do. Together, we're a network of medical professionals that handles anything and everything an athlete throws at us.

Parents reading this might think, *'Oh boy, that sounds expensive.'* I'm not saying you have to pay a squadron of doctors to follow your young athlete around every day from the time she picks up at racket as a toddler until she's in a professional jersey. I am suggesting, however, that a holistic approach requires more than one medical opinion and possibly multiple medical specialties. No single doctor is infallible; I'm certainly not, and I would distrust any doctor who claims to know everything.

A given athlete may require any number of combinations of treatments, both physical and psychological, to fully heal and return to their sport after an injury, or to stay healthy within it even without injuries. Don't be afraid to ask questions or get second opinions. The best doctors are already collaborating and won't be threatened if you seek help elsewhere.

Based on my years of experience in the field, I'd like to share some tips from our practice for parents seeking doctors, and for other medical professionals striving to treat, heal, and raise their own athletes.

EQUAL TREATMENT

Just as Bobby crafts a unique coaching plan for each athlete, so too do I examine and treat each patient with their own personal plan and it's true that my approach has been utilized by a number of elite athletes. That being said, there are many in my profession, especially those in the world of professional sports, who give special treatment to celebrity athletes or famous patients. Let me be blunt: I think that's crap.

It's important for parents to tell their kids that, no matter what their level of competition, they're equally deserving of love and attention. They should choose doctors who act in

> *It's important for parents to tell their kids that, no matter what their level of competition, they're equally deserving of love and attention.*

accordance with this teaching. Especially in the examination room, it doesn't matter if you're Tom Brady or a kid throwing the pigskin with his dad in the local park—you should get the same treatment.

Despite the fact that I specialize in sports medicine, my irreplaceable right-hand and office manager of 20 years, Carla Droege, doesn't know a thing about sports. I mean nothing. Many years ago, back when he was playing for the St. Louis Rams, Kurt Warner walked into my office for treatment. Some of our other staff were whispering and pointing, as you might when in the presence of a world-renowned, exceptionally talented athlete. Carla—partly because she didn't know who he was, and partly because this is just her personality—walked right up to Kurt and asked, "What do you want?"

She wasn't rude. She was just running the office and, on any given day in our waiting room, you could find a local farmer, next to a kid with no insurance from East St. Louis, next to a Hall-of-Famer or Olympian and they're prioritized only by their need for care and never by their notoriety. If you don't experience the same level of attention for your athlete as you see being given to others, it may be time to find better medical care.

HEAL FOR LIFE

In the same way that families should set their kids up for happiness in the long run, and coaches should train their players for success outside the court, I treat patients with an eye for the future. Yes, it's my job to get athletes back on the field and competing as quickly as possible, but I always prioritize their long-term safety and stability.

If I need to tell a parent or coach that their kid needs a month off of practice, despite their sometimes vehement protestations, I do it. Smart families know I'm looking out for their young athletes, and savvy coaches know that I'm considering, not just their chances in the playoffs, but their player's fatigue, nutrition, and emotional stability.

It doesn't matter if you're a weekend jogger or Jackie Joyner-Kersee—your long-term health is and should be the priority, and your chosen medical team should act accordingly. Maintaining this vital priority is another reason why communication between family, coach, and medical professionals is so important. All team members need to be open, honest, and trusting with one another in the service of raising the healthiest, happiest, fittest athletes we can. Working together, we not only get the athlete back onto the field faster, and for longer, but prevailingly, we're doing things right by the most important person of all—the athlete!

The Danger of Drugs

In my experience, if you gathered ten of the greatest Olympic athletes in the world and told them, *'Take steroids and you'll win a gold medal—but you'll die at 45,'* ten out of ten would say, *'Give me the steroids.'*

I can't tell you the number of times professional athletes have asked me about steroids. In these instances, it's my job to educate the athlete, and put them on a different path. Of course, I tell the athlete, "This is illegal;" "You'll lose this muscle mass the minute you stop with the pills or needles;" "We still don't know all the long-term negative effects of steroids;" and, "You'll end up hurting yourself."

I also remind my athletes that so many people—their teammates, families, and coaches—have put so much time, effort, and

> *I'd like to say this frank and truthful conversation always works . . . but—just as frankly—it doesn't.*

love into their lives, that turning to drugs is a pretty piss poor way to repay everyone. I'd like to say this frank and truthful conversation always works . . . but—just as frankly—it doesn't.

It's for that reason I'm including this section. Parents and coaches need to look out for their kids and players. Talk to them. Even recreational drugs like marijuana and alcohol are dangerous, especially to developing bodies and minds. Don't hesitate to connect with your athlete to put together a recovery plan you can work through as a team.

The following table outlines several substances commonly abused by athletes, including signs of abuse and long-term side effects.

Substance Being Used/ Abused	Common Reasons for Usage	Spotting the Signs of Abuse	(Some of the) Short- and Long-Term Side Effects
Steroids	Pressures related to having a bigger size and better performance athletically, ego and vanity (particular in men) based on the physical effects of usage	Rapid or unexplained increased muscle mass, paranoia, aggression, self-isolation, severe acne	High blood pressure, blood clots, heart attacks, stroke, artery damage, early male pattern baldness (men and women), enlarged breasts (in men), decreased breast size (in women), excessive bodily hair growth and voice deepening (women), decreased sperm production and shrunken testes (men), jaundice, oily skin, cysts, acne, permanent short stature (if taken in adolescence)

Substance Being Used/ Abused	Common Reasons for Usage	Spotting the Signs of Abuse	(Some of the) Short- and Long-Term Side Effects
Alcohol	Easily available, socially acceptable pain reliever and relaxer; often used in peer pressure situations	Grogginess, isolation, loss of interest in things he/she used to enjoy	Addiction more likely if large consumption occurs regularly before adulthood, liver problems, weight issues, emotional instability
Painkillers	Many pain killer addictions begin with OTC medications or even a legal prescription for a legitimate injury; high tolerance and easy availability make these drugs easy-to-turn-to fixes for the athlete	Drowsiness, mood-changes, weakness, nausea, dizziness, depression, itching, sweating	Severe withdrawal symptoms (vomiting, muscle and joint pains, diarrhea, cold flashes), highly addictive, agitation, constipation, slowed breathing and weakened cardiovascular activity
Sleeping Pills	Usually started to innocently battle exhaustion and adrenaline, easy over-the-counter availability, socially acceptable	Weakness, drowsiness	Insomnia, fatigue

Substance Being Used/ Abused	Common Reasons for Usage	Spotting the Signs of Abuse	(Some of the) Short- and Long-Term Side Effects
Aderall (or other ADD/ ADHD Medicine)	Lack of focus, need for productivity on short timelines, socially acceptable today, easily available	Anxiety, twitchy or involuntary movements, "scatter-brained" speaking, mood swings, emotional instability, nervousness	Vision problems, hallucinations, hostility, aggression, depression, suicide risk, impotence, photosensitivity, insomnia, heart attacks
Sudafed	While this easily available pseudo-ephedrine is used as a nasal decongestant, this drug is also a stimulant/upper that it is banned by the World Anti-Doping Agency	Insomian, dizziness, vomiting, addiction	Long-term use of the medication could result in fear, anxiety, convulsions, seizures, and hallucinations

Simply put, there is no such thing as benign drug usage. It can be career-ending for an athlete, and—for anyone—life-altering. When these drugs lead to even stronger addictions (and there are many books on those), they can cause irreparable physical, mental, and emotional damage and even kill.

The Unimaginable

Few things could kill a parent more than knowing that a trusted adult put into their child's life was not trusted at all and, in fact, should be one of the very people from whom the child was protected.

♦♦♦♦♦♦

Excerpt from "Larry Nassar: The Making of a Monster Who Abused Gymnasts for Decades" by Tim Evans (with Joe Guillen, Gina Kaufman, Marisa Kwiatkowski, Matt Mencarini, Mark Alesia, and IndyStar)[6]:

Over 15 years, longtime gymnastics coach Patrick Hulliung relied on (Dr. Larry) Nassar's recommendations for training methods that prevent injury. Hulliung attended the doctor's

---

[6] Author: Tim Evans "Larry Nassar: The Making of a Monster Who Abused Gymnasts for Decades." Wkyc.com, 8 Mar. 2018, www.wkyc.com/article/news/nation-now/larry-nassar-the-making-of-a-monster-who-abused-gymnasts-for-decades/465-695c82c5-ab9c-41d9-af65-7b2262b73311.

seminars, read his books, consulted with him about injuries and sent athletes to him for treatment.

Hulliung even invited Nassar to his gym, the World Class Gymnastics Center in Belleville, Ill., to screen athletes.

"Respect level for him was through the roof," said Hulliung. "He was the best."

Never, in all those years, did Hulliung hear a whisper of allegations against the famed doctor. There were rumors about coaches in the sport, sure. But not Nassar.

So Hulliung said he was horrified in January 2016 when [one of his athletes], a former gymnast whom he regarded as family, described in detail how Nassar had inserted his fingers into the most private areas of her body.

The medical appointment had happened five years earlier, when [Hulliung's gymnast] was suffering back pain as a senior [at University]. The [athlete] tried to justify Nassar's actions. Teammates told her they had experienced something similar. She called her mom, who argued something didn't sound right. [The gymnast] defended Nassar, but she said "the feeling of wrongdoing haunted my mom."

It was [the gymnast's] mother who prompted her to tell Hulliung and another coach while they were visiting each other in Florida.

Hulliung said he couldn't sleep that night. He felt guilty for being one of the people who recommended Nassar to [his athlete].

"I knew it was wrong from the moment she said it to me," he said.

But he hesitated. He wanted to give Nassar the benefit of the doubt. So, when he returned to Illinois days later, he met with his friend Dr. Richard Lehman, medical director for the U.S. Center for Sports Medicine in St. Louis.

Lehman said in a recent interview that the coach looked terrible. Hulliung relayed [the] story and asked Lehman what he thought about Nassar's techniques.

"In 33 years of this," Lehman said, "and, you know, going to a million meetings and hearing a million talks and reading the literature and kind of knowing everybody in sports medicine, I've really never heard of anything like this."

Lehman said he had never heard of a technique like that to treat back pain.

"That's just full-on sexual assault," Lehman told Hulliung. "I just can't put it any other way."

The coach hung his head.

"That's kind of my take on it as well," Hulliung replied.

"It was a grim discussion," Lehman said in an interview, "and it was grim for both of us."

◆◆◆◆◆◆

The world watched USA Gymnastics fall apart when its most prominent doctor, attached to the most prestigious programs in the country, including the Olympian factory Houston-based Károlyi Ranch, was found to have been committing sexual assaults on the young girls in his care for two decades. The toxic environment of winning at all costs had closed the eyes and ears of the adults who were trusted to care for some of the country's most elite female athletes. It was only the latest such scandal to rock the athletic world.

Sexual abuse toward children and adolescents is a stark reality worldwide. A common misperception about child sexual abuse is that it is a rare event perpetrated against girls by male strangers in poor, inner-city areas. To the contrary, child sexual abuse is a much-too-common occurrence that results in harm to millions of children, boys and girls alike, in large and small communities, and across a broad range of cultural and socioeconomic backgrounds. These acts are perpetrated by many types of offenders, including men and women, strangers, trusted friends or family, and people of all sexual orientations, socioeconomic classes, and cultural backgrounds[7].

In short, sexual abuse, as much as it's uncomfortable to recognize ugly facts, is not rare. In America, a sexual assault occurs every 73 seconds; one in six women has experienced some form of sexual assault; and one in every 33 men has been sexually assaulted or abused[8].

In athletics, the instances of sexual crimes are even higher than in the general population. According to the Journal of Clinical Sports Psychology, the sport environment has been recognized as a microcosm of sexual harassment and assault. The Jerry Sandusky[9] and Larry Nassar scandals of the past decade have illuminated the painful reality that child and adolescent athletes, in their tight knit, highly aspirational environments, are vulnerable to sexual misconduct by figures they emulate and trust[10].

---

[7] Murray, Laura K et al. "Child sexual abuse." Child and adolescent psychiatric clinics of North America vol. 23,2 (2014): 321-37. doi:10.1016/j.chc.2014.01.003

[8] "Scope of the Problem: Statistics." RAINN, www.rainn.org/statistics/scope-problem

[9] Former college football coach with Penn State found guilty in 2012 of sexually assaulting 10 boys over the course of 15 years using his position of power in football leadership

[10] Reel, Justine J., and Emily Crouch. "#MeToo: Uncovering Sexual Harassment and Assault in Sport." Journal of Clinical Sport Psychology, vol. 13, no. 2, 2019, pp. 177–179., doi:10.1123/jcsp.2018-0078.

Hulliung aches over the fact that he had athletes abused by Nassar, but he never wants the gymnasts he loves as family to feel guilt or shame.

The coach told me, "My athlete didn't want to be labeled as a victim number. We said, 'No. You're an athlete, and a name, and a person, not a number. No matter what happened, that doesn't define who you as an athlete or even who I am as a coach; it defines Dr. Nassar.'"

Nassar's crimes, though, or at least their persistence over the course of decades, could have been prevented[11]. When he finally went to trial in 2017, 204 women gave victim's statements. Some of them had been under the age of 13 when Nassar's assaults occurred . . . and some had reported him. In fact, numerous "trusted" adults knew about his actions. The fact that they didn't report him or protect our athletes does define who they are as leaders. The same was true of Jerry Sandusky who had sexually abused young boys years before him[12]. In the case of the latter, Joe Paterno and others in power were aware of Sandusky's abuses.

---

[11] Kozlowski, Kim. "What MSU Knew: 14 Were Warned of Nassar Abuse." Detroit News, The Detroit News, 19 Jan. 2018, www.detroitnews.com/story/tech/2018/01/18/msu-president-told-nassar-complaint-2014/1042071001/.

[12] Ganim, Sara. "CNN Exclusive: Joe Paterno May Have Known of Earlier Jerry Sandusky Abuse Claim, Police Report Reveals." CNN, Cable News Network, 11 Sept. 2017, www.cnn.com/2017/09/09/us/penn-state-paterno-sandusky-police-report.

The U.S. has been reactive in the area of sexual assault, rather than proactive, and that's just not good enough for our kids. It's wrong and we have to fix this. The cost is just too damned high not to!

♦♦♦♦♦♦

Physical abuse is usually visible. If kids are coming in multiple times with injuries that don't seem consistent with their sport, somebody is probably hurting that child. Then, it takes conversations and trust to get to the bottom of who that abuser might be. Is it a teammate? A coach, teacher, or leader in the child's life? A parent? Those conversations and investigations are difficult, but when open communications have been kept throughout the entire process of caring for the athlete, they can be had and there needs to be zero tolerance for the behavior.

Sexual abuse is a bit more clandestine. Not only does it not necessarily have a visible manifestation, but it's emotionally damaging and shameful for the victims, so they may work to hide the other signs. It's not their shame; but that's not how it feels to them. There are a few things that can be looked for. Loved ones may see that a great athlete suddenly begins coming home from events or practices feeling discouraged rather than energized, or a once-adored adult is ignored or avoided.

Often, we tend to chalk up drastic behaviors in our young people to the fact that they are teenagers going through puberty, but parents should trust their instincts and have the hard conversations. Sometimes, the questions about possible sexual abuse feel as strange to adults as they will to the young men and women hearing them, but we can't be afraid of discomfort. What could be prevented is far worse.

Occasionally, even a consensual, but improper relationship can be uncovered in this way. Especially top athletes in high school can idolize a young coach. Just because a consensual relationship is taking place, doesn't make it an allowable one and such improper conduct has the potential to cause long-lasting emotional damage. By having a team that is unafraid to ask questions, the athlete will learn what is and what is not acceptable, as well as how a trusted, and loving adult behaves.

In the case of doctors who perform physical examinations or procedures, there are a few simple considerations, as well. Parents should ensure that their child is comfortable, appropriately covered, and accompanied by a parent or same-gendered nurse or technician . . . at all times.

I can't say it enough. We can do better. We must.

I.njury and Illness Management

The Common Injuries

As a surgeon, I deal with a lot of bodies that are broken, but I tapped into my medical philosophy very early in my career. I wasn't tasked with just healing injuries; I'm tasked with healing people. This is a long-term game and healing for that game is determined by the patient. An athlete may desire healing for the sake of sports improvement. He or she may wish for healing to simply go on normally in life. Or, the person may wish to push through just to prove it's possible and that lesson will carry forward into the rest of his or her life's experiences.

When most people picture sports injuries, they think of hard hits, cringeworthy collapses, and tough tackles. Those certainly happen, but the most common breaks and breakdowns are much more subtle, the result of stress, strain, or repetitive movement without the benefit of recovery and therapy. Roughly 75 percent of the injuries we see at the U.S. Center for Sports Medicine fall into this latter category.

One of the most common injuries, especially in young athletes, is to the growth plate, the cartilaginous tissue at the end of long bones and, as you can see below, a young body has many of these potential injury zones. Growth plate injuries happen when specific muscles or bones are overworked, without ample opportunity for rest and recovery, or the cross-training and development of surrounding muscles. Fortunately, as with the majority of injuries I see, growth plate injuries are totally preventable.

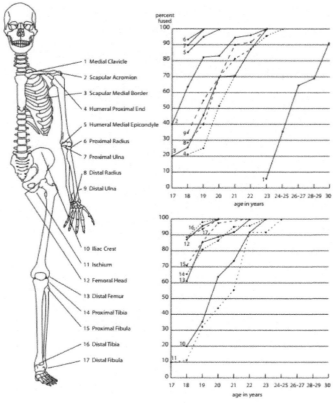

Pictured above: Growth plate locations and ages at which the bones are fully fused. Diagram Source: White, T. D., et al. Human Osteology. Academic, 2012.

In the earlier-provided age guide, I advocated for letting kids through age 12 to vary their sport involvement, rather than to specialize. The medical reason for that is growth plate injuries. These early years are very formative; if a young athlete repeats the same action over and over again—like shooting free throws without rest or pitching day after day without any time off—his muscles, bones, joints, and growth plates will suffer overuse and strain. This invariably leads to injury. As an example, when kids go from a school league, to a private league, to a recreation league, to a camp, to lessons, all focusing on the same sport, or—even worse—the same position, damage is being done that will hurt both the child's potential athletic prospects, as well as his or her lifelong physical health.

Cross country and long-distance runners who do not participate in other sports, for instance, sometimes suffer angular deformities in which the outside of the leg grows, but the inside does not. Pitchers may incur the same problem at the shoulder or elbow. These injuries are serious and, if not addressed (and prevented) early on, could require surgery in adulthood. Even once operated on, the athlete may have persistent arthritis, long-term pain, or even lifelong deformations. Giving kids a shot at multiple sports in their youth is a good way to keep them excited, engaged, and fit, while also reducing their likelihood of stress fractures or growth plate injuries and maintaining their long-term health.

You may think that you have the next Michael Jordan, but even Michael Jordan, himself, was cut from his middle school basketball team. What your child is doing in his or her sport before the age of 12 is not going to determine his or her future in athletics. Don't buy into the lie. Period. Give them a chance for more than sports; give them a chance for a long, healthy life.

♦ ♦ ♦ ♦ ♦ ♦

Let's look at other common stresses, strains, and injuries, as well as the treatments and surgeries required to correct them.

LITTLE LEAGUE ELBOW

Medial apophysitis or Little League Elbow, is a widening or breaking down of the growth plate. It's almost like a fracture, and can result in shorter limbs and angular joint deformities. Per the name, it's common among throwers, pitchers, and catchers. It occurs in our youngest athletes and is more common than tennis elbow, Tommy John, or rotator cuff injuries.

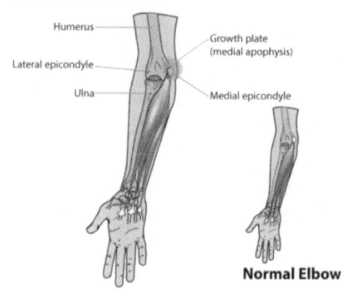

Humerus

Lateral epicondyle

Ulna

Growth plate
(medial apophysis)

Medial epicondyle

Normal Elbow

Source: sportsmd.com.

To prevent Little League Elbow, athletes first must rest appropriately. It seems simple, but most good things are. You'd be amazed by how many injuries go away, or can be prevented, by simply letting the body recover properly. Athletes must also train and strengthen the appropriate body parts and study proper pitching mechanics.

For parents and coaches, limit pitch counts. Let pitchers rest and recover. If the injury has already occurred, injections of platelet-rich plasma (PRP) or stem cells can help the tendons heal. Coaches should consult with kinesiologists and doctors on the biomechanics of pitching and throwing.

TENNIS OR GOLF ELBOW

Lateral epicondylitis, or tennis/golf elbow, is an overuse injury common among golfers, racquetball players, and tennis players. It usually strikes an athlete's lead, or dominant, arm, and frequently troubles older, rather than younger athletes.

With tennis/golf elbow, the outer tendons in the elbow become tender due to poor blood supply, making it difficult to grip or move the wrist. If left untreated, tendons can pull off the bone, which is very painful.

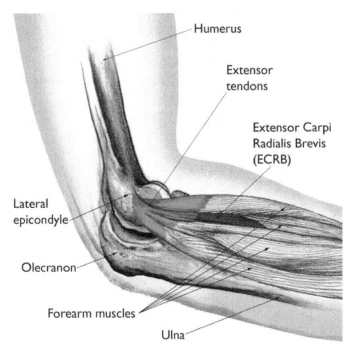

Source: The Body Almanac. © American Academy of Orthopedic Surgeons, 2003.

To prevent tennis/golf elbow, allow the athlete to rest and recover. For tennis players, take days where all you do is hit backhands or serves, and do conditioning or footwork. Try cross-training like swimming, weightlifting, or using resistance bands.

If pain persist, physical therapy and PRP are great options, with a 90 percent success rate in reducing pain and getting an athlete back on the court. Note that I'm sharing PRP as a recommendation once more and not the once-common cortisone shots. Ensure that your medical teams are on top of the latest recommendations for the best long-term health of your athlete.

As a last resort, there's a surgical alternative, which involves removing the damaged tendon and sewing the healthy bits of tendon back to onto the bone. Recovery time is three to six months, with physical therapy lasting up to a year.

ROTATOR CUFF INJURY

The rotator cuff is the confluence of muscles and tendons that attaches the arm to the chest. Rotator cuff injuries are common among athletes who lift or throw, notably pitchers, quarterbacks, soccer goalies, basketball players, volleyball players, and throwers in track and field.

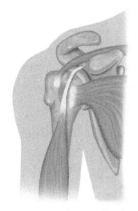
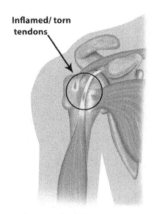

Inflamed/ torn
tendons

For treatment and prevention, rest the shoulder joint. Strengthen the rear deltoid, trapezius, and latissimus dorsi. Set limits to pitch counts and abide by them, study the throwing motion, and strengthen less-used parts of the body like pectorals and biceps. Physical therapy is a good option, as are injections of stem cells and PRP. Failing all that, we have to resort to surgery.

Arthroscopic surgery involves sewing tendons back onto the shoulder bone, as well as fixing injuries in the biceps tendon. It's painful and involves significantly limited mobility, sometimes for months, even with the best physical therapy and rehabilitation.

PATELLOFEMORAL PAIN SYNDROME

Patellofemoral pain is very common. Athletes who spend long periods of time squatting or jumping may suffer from it. It's more common in females than in males. The patella is the kneecap and the femur is the thigh bone; pain occurs when both are strained through overuse.

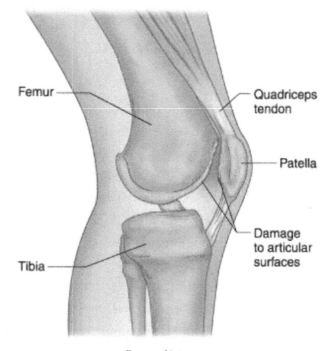

Source: kintec.net.

There are more than three million cases per year of patellofemoral pain syndrome. Rest alone will not fix the problem; most patients require some combination of rest, recovery, and physical therapy to fully heal.

Take pressure off the kneecap, stretch the iliotibial band, hamstrings, and hip flexors, and strengthen the vastus medialis obliques, hip abductors and adductors, and glutes.

Failing that, however, a patient may need cartilage reconstruction, a surgery that, though it has undergone many advancements, still may take three to six months from which to recover.

TOMMY JOHN

Tommy John is another name for the ulnar collateral ligament (UCL), the ligament that connects the bones of the arm (humerus, and ulna). Tommy John injury, most common among baseball pitchers, occurs in one of two ways. The UCL can fail slowly through repetitive stress, or it can rupture acutely, with a single hard pitch. Pitchers should watch for loss of velocity—the ligament is likely too thin and stretched out—followed by a loss of ball control— possibly a partial tear. When a ligament finally tears, pitchers experience a pop, then a tingling that is followed by pain after a hard throw or pressure pitch.

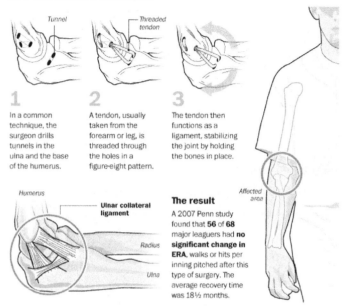

1 In a common technique, the surgeon drills tunnels in the ulna and the base of the humerus.

2 A tendon, usually taken from the forearm or leg, is threaded through the holes in a figure-eight pattern.

3 The tendon then functions as a ligament, stabilizing the joint by holding the bones in place.

The result

A 2007 Penn study found that **56 of 68** major leaguers had **no significant change in ERA**, walks or hits per inning pitched after this type of surgery. The average recovery time was 18½ months.

Source: Baseball Prospectus, American Journal of Sports Medicine | Bonnie Berkowitz and Alberto Cuadra/The Washington Post May 3, 2014

You can't necessarily avoid a Tommy John injury, but you can reduce your risk. Limit pitch counts, limit pressure pitches, incorporate full-arm rest days focused on cardio or leg training. Cross-train with yoga, swimming, or with resistance bands, and work to strengthen the core and posterior shoulder.

In the case of partial tearing, Dr. Stahle and I have seen great success with PRP and stem cell injections. Complete tears, though, will require surgery. Rehab after surgery will take three to four months, followed by a month or two of no-windup pitches.

Recovering athletes can start pitching again at four to five months, but it will take an additional three to four before they are able to return to full pitch counts, and even longer until they're back to full strength, high-speed pitches. For professional pitchers, this process usually takes nine to twelve months in total. While there have been exceptions, it's typically just not safe for the body to get there quicker.

ACL TEAR

The anterior cruciate ligament (ACL), the central ligament of the knee, stabilizes the knee against rotational stress. Tears are frequent among basketball, volleyball, soccer, and football players, as well as skiers. Tears are much more common among female athletes and are the most widespread knee injury among non-athletes.

The majority of ACL tears are acute, meaning they happen from deceleration or rotation. Athletes usually hear a pop; frequently, their teammates also hear the pop. There's intense pain and almost immediate swelling.

You can decrease the likelihood an ACL tear. Train with neuroproprioceptive exercises—go through jumping deceleration patterns and practice how to land (knees bent with a wide-legged stance). This kind of training should be standard among our young athletes.

Left knee bones in flexion (bent)

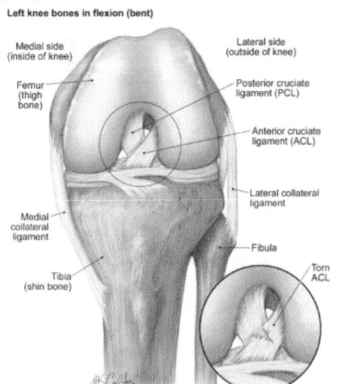

Source: Illustrator, MK Carlton. "Prevent ACL Injuries" from American Orthopedic Society for Sports Medicine. www.stopsportsinjuries.org.

Treatment of ACL tears has undergone a significant metamorphosis. Partial tears can improve with PRP or stem cell injections combined with physical therapy. This approach may work for athletic hobbyists, but for professionals or those with a full tear, surgery is the way to go.

Today, surgeons reconstruct the ACL with ligaments or tendons from other parts of the body and use synthetic fiber tape dipped in collagen to augment the new ligament. Return from surgery takes a bit longer, from nine to twelve months—with the special tape, the knee is a bit tighter—but you end up with a stronger, more fully recovered knee.

The key to recovery, though, truly is rehab. Athletes must have a good physical therapist. Listen to your therapist and do your exercises and stretches. Your surgery doesn't mean anything if you don't do the work required to get your joint back into proper shape. This is true with all surgeries, but it's particularly important with the ACL because you use it so often—every step you take—and there are so many potential pitfalls for regression and re-injury.

DISLOCATIONS

Dislocations—when a joint pops quickly out of its socket—are common, especially in wrestling and mixed martial arts. They also occur as a result of overthrowing, and in physical contact sports such as hockey and football. Dislocations range from fingers to elbows and knees, though shoulders are the most common.

A dislocated joint can typically be manipulated back into place—that's called reducing the joint. Many team trainers and coaches know how to do this. While the pain of reduction is immediate and sharp, it fades quickly. If a coach or trainer is not able to reduce the joint, the athlete must go to the emergency room. After initial treatment, the athlete should follow up with an orthopedic surgeon.

One of the big problems with dislocations is that the more they happen, the more likely it is that they'll happen again in the future. Watch out for repeat dislocations, especially in the shoulder. Recurring shoulder dislocations may be a sign of a more serious glenoid labrum tear, or a tear in the shoulder socket rim. If the athlete hears a clicking sound or feels like her arm is getting caught or stopped while throwing, consult a doctor immediately.

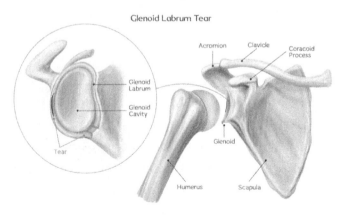

Source: REHAB, from MyPatient.com

As far as treatment, for someone with a one-time dislocation, physical therapy, strengthening, PRP, and stem cell injections can be sufficient. For someone with repeated dislocations, surgical reconstruction is the only answer.

PATELLAR INSTABILITY

The patella, or kneecap, is another commonly dislocated joint. The joint commonly dislocates to the outside—or laterally—which is very painful. This is called patellar instability. Pain usually diminishes after the joint has been reduced. Dislocation is common in dancers, soccer players, and other agile athletes, though it can happen to anyone. It's quite common, unfortunately.

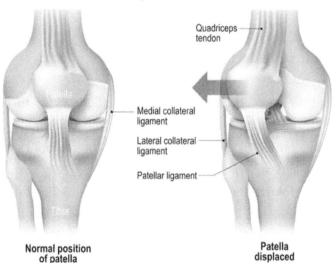

Source: healthjade.net.

Most first-time dislocations can be treated with physical therapy, PRP, stem cell injections, and knee braces. Athletes suffering multiple dislocations will likely require surgery, which involves repairing the medial patellofemoral ligament (MPFL) and addressing any other damage done to the joint.

SPRAINS

Sprains are a general term for a ligament injury. They are graded zero to three with three being a complete tear. They're most common at the ankle and can usually be treated at home with rest, ice, compression, and elevation. Over-the-counter (OTC) pain medicine such as ibuprofen can help, as well. For less severe sprains, physical therapy works well. Grade three sprains may require surgery.

FRACTURES

When a bone breaks, it's called a fracture. Fractures are very common. The most commonly broken bone is the clavicle, followed by the bones in the hand or wrist.

Most fractures are caused by collisions or falls. Proper pads, personal safety equipment, playing surfaces and fields with some give, and safe playing rules can all lessen the risk of broken bones, but it's impossible to prevent them entirely.

If there's only a crack in the bone, that's a non-displaced fracture, which can be treated with a cast. If there's a full break in the bone, or the bones dislocate, that's a displaced fracture. If the bone pokes through the skin, that's an open fracture, which is the most dangerous because of the increased risk of infection.

For a minimally displaced fracture, recovery time is two to three weeks. For a fully displaced fracture, it can be four to six weeks. If the injury requires surgery, the recovery time can be months.

CAULIFLOWER EAR

Cauliflower ear is the result of direct trauma to the cartilage of the ear. If blood pools in the ear and is not allowed to drain, the cartilage contracts and deforms, leaving a shriveled appearance. Other symptoms are loss of hearing, tinnitus, and persistent headaches. This happens most commonly in wrestling, boxing, and mixed martial arts.

Wearing headgear is the best way to prevent cauliflower ear, but the injury can also result from pressure, not just contact.

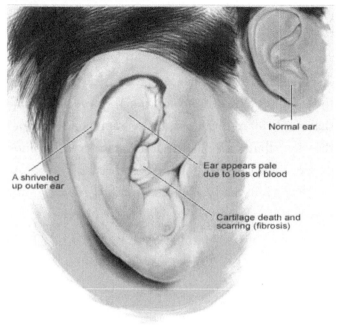

Source: *medicinenet.com.*

CONCUSSIONS

Football is, of course, most well-known for its high incidence of concussions, but they're quite prevalent in hockey, lacrosse, and other contact sports. In soccer, heading a ball can lead to brain trauma, especially in young, still-developing females.

In football, concussions and injury more broadly are exacerbated by the fact that leagues are organized based on age, not size. That means you could have a 100-pound fourteen-year-old lining up against a 250-

pound eighteen-year-old. This just isn't right. And, counterintuitively, kids recover slower from concussions than adults, so this is a particularly nasty problem in youth football. This issue is well-documented so I won't say more on the subject, except that all parents should consider whether it's really worth risking their kid's future health to play a sport, and—if it is—then please help your kid be as safe as they can be and advocate for proper equipment and safe play within their sports and leagues.

HEAD INJURIES

There are multiple kinds of head injuries. A concussion, obtained as described above, is a mild or moderate traumatic brain injury (TBI). Players who suffer concussions often report feeling like they're unfocused, or in a fog, but they are otherwise neurologically intact. They should exit the game immediately, seek medical evaluation in a day or two, and usually abstain from sports for one to two weeks (minimum). Don't cheat this timeline.

Other TBIs are much more severe. For example, an epidural hematoma is a blood clot underneath the skull (but on top of the covering that surrounds the brain). A person who has suffered an epidural hematoma may lose consciousness, vomit, seize, or deteriorate neurologically. This is a medical emergency; the person needs to go to the emergency room via ambulance immediately.

(Repetitive) Head Traumas

Finally, and I mean finally as in it took decades to get here, there's repetitive head traumas that are non-concussive. This is perhaps the most dangerous of the three types of head traumas because they build up—unchecked—over time. The kid who takes the hard hit is looked at, maybe even brought to the emergency room. But the kid who takes a dozen milder hits that he walks away from? We don't think twice about it. That's just the game; it's physical. We may even take some pride in the kid's toughness.

If you hit a person thirty times and it's not a concussion, but thirty-consecutive pre-concussive hits, those aren't free. There is no such thing as a non-violent blow . . . to one's head. The hit may not create a concussion or a hematoma, but a season of them adds up and a career of them could be deadly.

Brain trauma isn't necessarily associated with a concussion. This is some of the ugliness that we've ignored for decades. It's not that we didn't know it. It's too much common sense and logic to not know that repeatedly hitting somebody in the head will mess with that person's brain. So, we knew. We just ignored it and we still don't have a fully-proven way to measure it. We do know, unfortunately, when we autopsy a dead brain, that it's all screwed up. What good does that do for the athlete, though?

This type of trauma is seeing an uptick in soccer athletes, including women who are growing more aggressive in the sport and performing more headers. It also presents in rugby players and hockey athletes. However, it is football that has the systemic issue that we can no longer ignore.

At the age of 43, Junior Seau committed suicide via a gunshot to his chest. He didn't want to hurt his brain because he wanted it left for autopsy and study. The passionate Hall-of-Fame linebacker had been on All-Pro and Super Bowl teams over an outstanding almost twenty-year professional career in the NFL.

The National Institute of Health (NIH), upon studying his brain, concluded that Seau suffered from chronic traumatic encephalopathy (CTE). CTE leads to memory loss, confusion, dementia, rage—which sometimes is outwardly focused and results in violence—and depression. CTE is believed to be the result of repetitive head trauma and it has taken the extreme and desperate brain-saving suicide measures of hurting and broken NFL retirees, like Seau, to open the eyes of the world to the condition. He's one of at least six who are known to have taken their own lives—while preserving their brains—including 21-year-old Washington State University quarterback

Tyler Hilinski, who had CTE and, according to autopsy results, the brain of a 65-year-old.

Thankfully, not all of those whose brains were studied took their own lives, but many of them suffered greatly and, only after their deaths, could CTE be diagnosed. These are men who were our heroes. They become very depressed and aware of their being screwed up, but they didn't have any answers for improving their conditions.

I have seen some of these guys in my practice. And when you couple the condition they have with the reality of an NFL career length, you end up with someone who's not even 30 who allowed his body and head to be beaten up for entertainment, and now he's on medications and has to have medical care, possibly for the rest of his life. He has depressive disorders and uncontrollable violent urges.

These guys don't see a way out.

When neuropathologist, Dr. Ann McKee examined the brains of 111 deceased former NFL players, it was found that 110 of them suffered from the maddening CTE condition[13] . . . more than 99 percent!

---

[13] *Ward, Joe, et al. "111 N.F.L. Brains. All But One Had C.T.E." The New York Times, The New York Times, 25 July 2017, www.nytimes.com/interactive/2017/07/25/sports/football/nfl-cte.html*

It doesn't matter how great the sport of football is—we can't allow this to keep happening. I'll admit, I love football; but the doctor, and—more importantly—the human in me, knows that this can't go on. I won't be surprised if, in the future, we see either a radically different version of American football, or no football at all.

The Illnesses

While injuries are acute and typically easy to diagnose, a number of illnesses can commonly present in athletes, as well. Some of these illnesses come on quickly and others are recognized through examination and knowing what to look for. Athletes, of course, can experience all of the same illnesses as non-athletes, but they may be more susceptible to a handful that I've seen in my years of practice.

THERMOREGULATION ISSUES

In sports, it is typically heat, and not cold, that can be dangerous. If it's 100 degrees outside and you're six foot six and 320-pounds, running around in full football gear, that's not safe. Players who compete in these conditions may suffer heat disease which includes cramps, heat exhaustion, heat stroke, and even death. Coaches should know better than to have such workout scenarios and parents should speak up for the protection of their children if these unsafe conditions are present for practices.

Usually, an athlete begins by feeling hot. Then he begins excessive sweating, before generally feeling "not right" or nauseous. The last phase of heat disease is when the athlete stops sweating. It may seem like a good sign; but the opposite is true. The body has stopped regulating for heat. That's when cramps, confusion, and seizures can set in. Coaches should always be aware of safe conditions, have water handy; and be willing to call practice off, or change to an indoor workout if players are getting ill or weather does not safely permit practice.

The last phase of heat disease is when the athlete stops sweating. It may seem like a good sign; but the opposite is true.

It's not just football players: tennis players, soccer players, cross-country runners—anyone competing outside is vulnerable. For those suffering from heat exhaustion in any form, help them get inside and cool them off. Don't hold practice at the hottest time of day—usually three or four o-clock in the afternoon. Replace electrolytes and calories, not just water. And remember that practice does not have to be long in order to be effective.

ASTHMA

Exercise-induced asthma is common. Young athletes who have it will wheeze and have difficulty breathing, and this usually starts right after or even during activity, which itself causes the asthma. Jackie Joyner-Kersee had asthma, for instance, usually brought on by the famously taxing 800-meter run.

Exercise-induced asthma is usually medicated with an inhaler. Most kids hit the inhaler, feel better, and are good to go. If an athlete's asthma is not exercise-related, it's important to include medical professionals in conversations about the safety of the athlete participating in sports. Asthma is not a death sentence to athletics, but awareness and adjustment can ensure that the athlete is safe.

CONTACT ILLNESSES AND ISSUES

A traumatic hematuria is caused by direct contact with the kidney or back. Athletes suffering from this may use the bathroom and discover blood in their urine or stool. Sometimes, a fractured rib will puncture a kidney. Other times, it's just a deep bruise. Either way, the athlete needs to see a doctor.

Much more severe is commotio cordis. This rare, almost freak condition occurs when someone is hit in the chest with a ball, hockey stick, puck, elbow, or leg, and simply dies. The hit is hard enough and in exactly the wrong place, and it either stops the heart or sends it into a malignant rhythm, resulting in death.

Properly protect your athlete with pads, on the side and in front to help prevent such mortal injuries.

But we can do more.

It's becoming more and more common for venues and facilities to require defibrillators. In the case of commotio cordis, if the victim receives a defibrillator shock, their risk of mortality goes from 100 to 43 percent. For every second saved, that risk goes down. Defibrillators are expensive, but nothing is worth someone dying from playing a sport. Organizations need to make this equipment mandatory in the facilities and locations where our young people play.

MONONUCLEOSIS

Mono, also called the kissing disease, is a virus common among teenagers and college-age athletes. It's highly contagious and runs rampant through teams. Symptoms include fever, swollen lymph nodes (especially in the neck and armpits), sore throat, and possible rash or spots. It can feel a lot like strep throat.

If untreated, mono can lead to enlargement of the spleen. A ruptured spleen can then result in death. That said, like most viruses, mono can be treated with hydration, antibiotics, and rest. Recovery takes time, but it is vital. Get to the doctor; start treatment; rest; and get back to life.

DEEP VEIN THROMBOSIS

Deep vein thrombosis—when blood clots form and travel to the lungs or heart—is often associated with older or sedentary adults, but it can happen to younger athletes, too. If the clot is not treated and dislodges directly to the heart or lungs, it can be fatal.

Athletes are vulnerable if, while traveling to road games, they must remain seated for long stretches of time, particularly if they're dehydrated or recently recovering from surgery. Usually, there is pain or discomfort. Ultimately, athletes need to be attuned to how their body feels and vocal with their team members—families, coaches, and doctors—if something feels off.

PTSD AND ANXIETY

Athletes suffering from post-traumatic stress disorder (PTSD) should see a psychiatrist or psychologist. Those who have suffered a number of concussions are more likely to have comorbid psychological issues like PTSD and anxiety. Such an athlete will have trouble getting back onto the field. The best treatment is to let them fully recover; don't force them to return to competition. "Get back on the horse," is a dated and potentially damaging method for managing this very real psychological issue. They'll come back when they're ready.

PTSD-related anxiety can be psychological, and the athlete should see a sports psychologist when this condition becomes known. While an athlete may have external factors that have nothing to do with sports, there are also some common reasons anxiety and PTSD can come from sports, directly.

In an athlete who's had a number of concussions, we might see this issue. That athlete should be removed from the field of play. Their impairment may be reflected in any number of areas in their life: school, relationships, work, home, and interpersonal interactions.

If anxiety remains untreated on the fields and courts of sports, it will leak into other aspects of the athlete's world. Also, If the young man or woman learns to manage the condition in sports, those lessons will carry into life. Remember that counselors are just as important as surgeons on the athlete's team of medical professionals.

◆◆◆◆◆◆

Overuse and traumatic injuries, as well as short- and long-term physical and emotional illnesses in athletes, go well beyond these pages, as do the preventions, treatments, and recoveries of such ailments. I've tried to touch on some of the most common concerns across these areas, but of course there are more. I haven't provided great detail on arthroscopic procedures, congenital disorders, vaccine-preventable illnesses, and more. It is vital to have a team of observant coaches, engaged family, and informed medical professionals to manage the unique situations each athlete may face.

After decades at the top echelon of orthopedic surgery and sports medicine, the amount of information my team and I have experienced can't begin to fit into these pages. You are welcome to visit our website at **uscenterforsportsmedicine.com** to read our blog, listen to the latest medical discoveries shared in the media, learn recovery protocols, and discover treatments for the injuries and illnesses from these pages and beyond. Hundreds of articles, cases, and descriptions are available as free information to better understand and manage the health and wellness of athletes from a medical perspective.

Not all injury and illness can be avoided in sports, but not all injury and illness can be avoided in the rest of life, either. Sports are a microcosm of that life. Let's help to ensure they reflect the very best we want to see in the long, healthy existences our children lead beyond athletics. Let's give our kids the tools they need to be better mentally, emotionally, physically, and relationally for all of their days.

The Scales

For athletic hobbyists, or those who don't exercise recreationally, being overweight is a common problem. Top athletes have body fat percentages in the single digits; most Americans sit in the 30 to 50 percent range. This is a big problem in the U.S. Parents, coaches, and medical staff can help. Parents and coaches can be frank but supportive with their kids.

Dr. Stahle deals with this sensitive topic by setting realistic goals. He tells overweight patients, "This is your weight now. And this is where you're supposed to be. You don't have to get there right away. All you have to do is lose one pound by time I see you in two weeks."

Stahle also prescribes exercise in the right way. An overweight person doesn't need to jump straight to marathons; taking the stairs or parking at the back of the parking lot are a start. It's important to encourage people. If your body mass index (BMI) is high as a teenager, your chance of maintaining a normal healthy weight for the rest of your life is less than one percent. We must all do our part to raise athletes, and humans, with healthy bodies meant to be maintained for long lives.

For a pre-pubescent child, there are a few caloric standards, but—as you can see from this chart from the Mayo Clinic[14], the standards are also about eating the right things, not just the right amount.

Ages 2 to 3: Daily guidelines for girls and boys

Calories	1,000-1,400, depending on growth and activity level
Protein	2-4 ounces
Fruits	1-1.5 cups
Vegetables	1-1.5 cups
Grains	3-5 ounces
Dairy	2 cups

---

[14] Staff, Mayo Clinic. "What Nutrients Does Your Child Need Now?" Mayo Clinic, Mayo Foundation for Medical Education and Research, 23 May 2020, www.mayoclinic.org/healthy-lifestyle/childrens-health/in-depth/nutrition-for-kids/art-20049335.

Ages 4 to 8: Daily guidelines for girls

Calories	1,200-1,800, depending on growth and activity level
Protein	3-5 ounces
Fruits	1-1.5 cups
Vegetables	1.5-2.5 cups
Grains	4-6 ounces
Dairy	2.5 cups

Ages 4 to 8: Daily guidelines for boys

Calories	1,200-2,000, depending on growth and activity level
Protein	3-5.5 ounces
Fruits	1-2 cups
Vegetables	1.5-2.5 cups
Grains	4-6 ounces
Dairy	2.5 cups

Ages 9 to 13: Daily guidelines for girls

Calories	1,400-2,200, depending on growth and activity level
Protein	4-6 ounces
Fruits	1.5-2 cups
Vegetables	1.5-3 cups
Grains	5-7 ounces
Dairy	3 cups

Ages 9 to 13: Daily guidelines for boys

Calories	1,600-2,600, depending on growth and activity level
Protein	5-6.5 ounces
Fruits	1.5-2 cups
Vegetables	2-3.5 cups
Grains	5-9 ounces
Dairy	3 cups

Ages 14 to 18: Daily guidelines for girls

Calories	1,800-2,400, depending on growth and activity level
Protein	5-6.5 ounces
Fruits	1.5-2 cups
Vegetables	2.5-3 cups
Grains	6-8 ounces
Dairy	3 cups

Ages 14 to 18: Daily guidelines for boys

Calories	2,000-3,200, depending on growth and activity level
Protein	5.5-7 ounces
Fruits	2-2.5 cups
Vegetables	2.5-4 cups
Grains	6-10 ounces
Dairy	3 cups

◆ ◆ ◆ ◆ ◆ ◆

Athletes, because they are generally fit, are more likely to face the opposite problem of becoming potentially underweight or over-obsessive about their exercise. With the exception of a handful of positions in the NFL, overweight is the less common problem in sports.

If someone comes in who has six or seven percent body fat, and he's very fit with good cardiovascular activity, he might actually be okay. There may be high muscle mass and therefore the athlete's BMI is not reflective in their health. Where health problems related to being underweight come in are in the unrealistic standards set within certain sports.

Where health problems related to weight come in are in the unrealistic standards set within certain sports.

Men have some sports that encourage poor eating habits. For example, wrestlers who wish to make weight and cut a great number of pounds to be in a lower weight class have been known to not eat for days at a time in an attempt to make weight. This is very unhealthy.

Female athletes face similar struggles when they are pushed to drop weight for faster speeds and when that weight drop is accomplished in unhealthy manners. One of the biggest issues in young female athletes is known as the female triad: low energy availability, low bone density, and amenorrhea.

Low energy availability (also called Relative Energy Deficiency Syndrome, or RED-S) is the result of insufficient nutrition. It's all about calories, protein, and proper nutrition. Top athletes train like fiends. They spend two to three hours on the track or the court. Then they lift. Then they repeat. To keep that up, you need a lot of calories; the 2000 calories a day being consumed by their non-athlete peers won't cut it for their lifestyle. Coaches and nutritionists must work with the athlete to make sure she has enough energy.

Low bone density in female athletes is also about insufficient nutrition. Vital nutrients strengthen and thicken the bones during a woman's younger, growing years. It's critical to build strong bones because, as early as age twenty-five, women lose around one percent of bone density per year. If you don't start out with strong bones to begin with, you'll be in trouble later in life; bone density affects everything from arthritis to childbearing.

Amenorrhea is the cessation of menstruation. It's one thing for a young woman to miss a period when starting on a new training regimen. It's another to continually miss them because that young woman is training too hard or not eating properly. I've seen track athletes brag about not having a period in three years. It may seem like a point of pride to show the hard work being put in on training and practice. What they may not realize, though, is that prolonged amenorrhea can permanently damage a woman's reproductive system.

Then there are eating disorders, things like anorexia, bulimia, and exercise bulimia. Society puts enormous pressure on us to look a certain way, and when you combine that with the pressure to hone the perfect athletic instrument—the body—you find young women and some young men with unhealthy relationships to eating and nutrition.

"If you're 10 years old and all you hear is, 'You're too heavy, you're too heavy,' what's a better recipe for an eating disorder?" Hulliung says, of young female athletes. *"Of course they have eating disorders; we've trained them to be bulimic and anorexic! Coaches in gymnastics especially have been complicit."*

Malnourishment, especially in females, can lead to stress fractures. In bulimia, when a person binge-eats and then forces vomiting, stomach acid may also destroy teeth and dissolve mouth tissue. Exercise bulimia, incidentally, is when one binges on exercise, well beyond their available energy or their body's healthy ability. Persistent anorexia and bulimia, in a twist of cruel irony, can actually lead to bloating (which only encourages the behavior further).

It can be an uncomfortable medical communication, but the female triad is a real problem. It's my responsibility for athletes to have a good body when they're done playing. And that means a good body internally, too. It's not a short-term game. I want the athletes I treat to have the option to have kids. They may choose not to, and that's fine, but I don't want to take that away from them while they are still young.

It's important for sports medicine physicians to have the hard conversations, be responsible for the long haul, and educate the whole team of the athlete, regardless of whether that is family, coaches, additional medical professionals such as nutritionists and gynecologists, or the athlete, herself.

If calorie-shorting is intentional or caused by an eating disorder, a psychologist or psychiatrist should be a part of the recovery equation. When an athlete is seeking only to lose weight, rather than to meet her energy needs, it could be a sign of an eating disorder. Untreated eating disorders are the equivalent of starvation; they ultimately lead to fatal heart or organ failure.

> *If an athlete is seeking only to lose weight, rather than to meet her energy needs, it could be the sign of an eating disorder.*

According to the American Psychiatry Association, there are a few other signs the team of an athlete should look for in order to recognize anorexia or bulimia.

Disorder	Causes	Symptoms	Treatment
Anorexia (Nervosa) – *Diagnosed when patients are 15 percent underweight*	Thoughts and emotions including perfectionism, low self-esteem, poor or distorted body image, "feeling fat," seeing oneself as overweight, and a fear of gaining weight. The two eating disorders often occur together.	Female triad, dry or yellowing skin, brittle hair and nails, anemia, constipation, low blood-pressure or pulse, shallow breaths, low body temperature, lethargy, and depression.	Interrupt binge-purge cycles (bulimia), psychotherapy to understand thought- and emotion-triggers, nutritional counseling, and general medical care to restore physical well-being.
Bulimia (Nervosa) – *Diagnosed through symptoms or when binge-purge cycles are witnessed*		Sore throat, swollen glands producing a "chipmunk-face" appearance, acid reflux, tooth decay, intestinal or kidney problems, and dehydration.	

When an athlete seeks to learn more about nutrition and caloric intake as part of her training, or when she is working to improve energy and performance, a caloric deficiency in that scenario would most likely be the result of applying misinformation. Proper communication and education can help those female athletes discover their true nutritional needs to stop RED-S in its tracks.

Whether the athlete needs better nutrition education, or more serious help to deal with eating disorders, the conversation needs to change from the top down when it comes to weight. Nothing is as important as the health of our children's bodies; not appearances, or a few less pounds to carry down a track. Parents, coaches, and medical staff must have open conversations with their sons and daughters about what is healthy, and what is dangerous.

The media creates significant disillusionment for young women and men, often leading athletes to a mix of undereating, over exercising, or misused medications such as laxatives to lose weight or steroids to gain muscle. The medical team, parents, and coaches need to be on-guard.

The issue of weight goes well beyond the scales. Healthy weight in athletes, as well as the perception of it in sports performance and media portrayal, is a much more complex picture than just looking at weight, body mass index, or body fat percentages. Doctors should consider the young man's or woman's metabolism, the athlete's heart health and blood pressure, and his or her overall fitness levels including strength, endurance, flexibility, agility, balance, and coordination, as well as his or her strong mental state and self-image.

Let us start seeking the answers to healthy weight. They come from a combination of exams and tests, observation and awareness of the athlete's team, and from both routine and more difficult and uncomfortable conversations.

S.egue to Life After Sports

The Transition

As shared when looking at realistic expectations and career-lengths, there will be athletes who "make it" to the big games of their sports. If their teams of family, coaches, and medical professionals do their jobs right, those young people will have a long healthy life left to continue living after their playing days are done.

So, what comes next?

Sports build drive into people and if that drive doesn't have somewhere to go after sports, the former athlete can feel lost, directionless, purposeless, or depressed. These conditions can be treated with psychological help, but—more importantly—they can be prevented with planning!

While the athlete is still involved in his or her athletic career, he or she should continue to learn, participate in activities and service, and experience events and hobbies outside of his or her sport. Exposure to other activities is the only way to know if there is interest and, even better, passion for something other than sports.

130

Sometimes that interest will run adjacent to athletic endeavors such as coaching, managing camps, speaking or writing about the sport, representing athletes in their finances and artistic endeavors, working in nutrition, or—as happened with me and Dr. Stahle—learning to treat and care for athletes rather than competing alongside them.

"I grew up on an Iowa City farm. My parents are mad I wasn't a farmer! I told my dad, 'I'm not smart enough to be a farmer. I don't know how to make tools, rotate crops, and run a farm business.'"

"My mom asked, 'Who's gonna take over the farm?'"

"'I don't know, mom, but not me.' I said."

"My little brother, who also works as an electrician, took it over."

"I wanted to be a Cubs second baseman. It took me just one professor in college to say, 'What are you going to do when you graduate?'"

"I told him, 'What do you mean? I'm gonna play baseball.'"

"'Maybe you should look at some other things,' he said."

"He looked at my grades and suggested medicine.

I was really good in biology. After a few meetings, I took the MCATS and it all clicked, but I still wanted to do sports medicine, specifically. I wanted to be around athletes. It's in my blood."

"I love the farm. I love baseball. But I couldn't do anything else but be a doctor."

(Dr. Steven Stahle)

Other times, the next career could be completely unrelated, but many of the skills that an athlete takes from sports could help him or her to make that next dream come true. Real estate and sales are both popular second careers that capitalize on the charisma and competition developed through sports. Media, journalism, advertising, and entertainment can also be transitions that take advantage of one's status. Sometimes, the athlete served in a charitably capacity as part of his or her team and a desire is born to help that cause after professional sports. The bottom line is that an athlete's passion needs to find an outlet in life when that outlet can no longer be his or her sport.

"I really wanted to go back to serve in East St. Louis. I had a desire to do good in the home community. We were taught to humble ourselves to come back. It's easy to walk away because you reached greatness, but someone thought of you and gave you their time. You didn't get there alone."

"I grew up coming through The Mayor Brown Community Center. It really impacted my life, not just in track and field, but working with the librarian and the senior citizens doing Meals on Wheels. I was introduced to sports through the community center. They were part of my extended family there. Everyone knew everyone. It was located in the park. I joined the team. My sister and neighbors near the park made up the team."

"When I went off to college, I lost my mom to meningitis. I came home and went straight to the Mayor Brown Community Center. I wanted love and people to embrace me and lift me up; instead, I was greeted with padlocks."

"'Where do the young people go now?' I thought."

"My goal as a freshman in college became putting that place back into the community . . . I didn't even know you needed money to open the center."

"When I made the Olympic team in 1984, I was still thinking about the center. After my second Olympics in 1988, I was able to have the time to start the journey. Eight years later, after raising funds in churches and through great people like Doc Rick, in 1996, I finished raising the funds."

"I opened the Jackie Joyner-Kersee Community Center in the year 2000. It was a 19-year dream! But thousands of kids have come through since."
(Jackie Joyner-Kersee)

There is life after sports and, while our athletes are in their careers, we can help them to build toward that life. We can prepare them socially, financially, holistically, and with an eye toward their next chapters' dreams and passions. Perhaps Coach Fennoy said it best:

> *"I love being a coach. There is such a chemistry between coaches and kids. I had that feeling from coaches when I was young, and I wanted to share it with the next generation. I wasn't going to be a professional in sports, so I went to school to teach. I was an educator first; I spent 11 years teaching physical education in East St. Louis and I practiced at being a coach at the elementary and intramural levels. Teaching and coaching were the sparkle for me."*

> *"With the right forums, students are able to discover what they are good at . . . through sports. You see the sparkle in their eyes when they're trying to figure themselves out. You put challenges before them and you see them achieve. That's bigger than when they medal."*

> *"Everything we did together had to be about the moment we were in. What were we doing together at a specific time? What was being achieved and celebrated? That was where relationship came from. I tapped into my internal love of sports, and that's what I wanted to teach them. It wasn't the sports, it was the LOVE."*

> *(Coach Nino Fennoy)*

E.njoy the Game

The "Play"

"**T**here are points in an Ironman[15] *when you hate what you're doing in that moment. It's a bad moment and you think, 'I never want to do this again,'*" said triathlete Louis DiGuiseppe. "*Then, you come down the chute and people are screaming and it's worth it. You went to the well and back . . . psychologically, physically, and emotionally. You cross the line and you can't wait to do it again. Despite all the race challenges and the misery you felt, you persevered and it's cool. It's really cool. I still get emotional about it.*"

◆ ◆ ◆ ◆ ◆ ◆

This may surprise you following the many things I believe need to be fixed in raising our athletes, but I hold firm to the belief that, when it comes to sports,

---

[15] Ironman is the top race length for triathlons. An Ironman triathlete must complete a 2.4 mile open-water swim, followed by a 112-mile bike ride, and a 26.2-mile marathon run. The majority The Ironman World Championship is held in Kona, Hawaii every year for athletes who qualify through other race events.

LET THEM PLAY! The essential word "play" is what most needs to come back. In that play, we have a platform by which we can build incredible young men and women who will have long, healthy, and productive lives. Athletic endeavors carry us far from the finish lines of the actual events and games. Many principles of sports are compelling in life:

- Discipline
- Teamwork
- Obligation
- Responsibility
- Self-Image
- Strength
- Health
- Time Management
- Confidence
- Multi-tasking
- Clean Living
- Goal Setting
- Self-betterment
- Adaptability
- Mental Toughness
- Pushing Your Limits
- Earning Success
- Listening
- Respecting Others
- Honor

I don't want to cheat the next generation of these invaluable skills that can be reinforced through sports. So, yes. LET THEM PLAY! If they happen to make a career in professional sports, we will cheer for them from the sidelines when this long pandemic season has passed, and those sidelines are open to the fans once more. But—if they don't—we damned well better cheer anyway as they become doctors, and fathers, and teachers, and philanthropists, and mothers, and workers, and our neighbors, and our friends. We need to remember that they can be better for having been athletes even if sports weren't their ticket into adulthood.

My friend Frank Cusumano, who works as a sportscaster with KSDK in St. Louis, has been courtside for the Final Four and trackside for the Kentucky Derby. He's worked at the World Series, the Super Bowl, and at Olympic-level track events. He told me that none of it came close to watching his own three children in action in sports. He didn't miss many shots over the years, or at-bats. He got to watch his daughter and two sons in basketball, one of his own first loves. He also supported them in golf and baseball.

Frank's oldest, Alex, led Loyola to an NCAA Golf final. He asked Frank once after a tournament, "Dad, do you pray for my success when I'm out there?"

Frank said, "Well, what did you shoot today?"

"72," Alex answered.

"Then, I prayed 72 times," his dad said.

I'm guessing you've never heard of the great golfer Alex Cusumano. But that moment mattered, not just for an NCAA final, but for the bond between a father and son. What moments that matter are waiting for you and your child? LET THEM PLAY!

"I'll keep doing it until Dr. Rick says I'm done."
(Louis DiGuiseppe)

The Memories

Medicine in the Media — I've been lucky to talk sports medicine and orthopedics on Fox 2, KMOX, KSDK Channel 5, the Charlie Tuna Show, with friend Frank Cusumano, on the "Ask Dr. Rick" show, in print publications, and throughout the media.

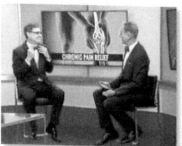
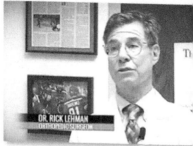

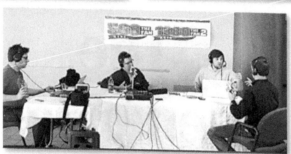

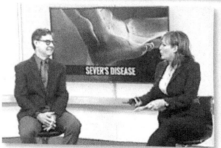
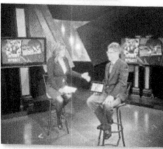

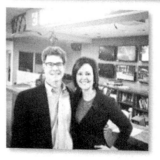

Top to bottom, left to right: Fox 2 interview with John Pertzborn on joint health—January 2020; KSDK 5 interview breaking down the Vladimir Tarasenko shoulder injury; live broadcasting with AM 590 "The Fan"; Fox 2 Now interview on Sever's Disease, Fox 2 Now interview segment; in the studio with Sara Dayley (Ken Dayley's daughter) before an on-air interview.

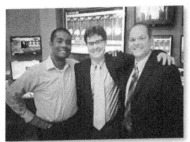
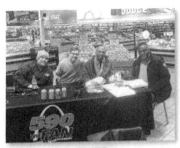
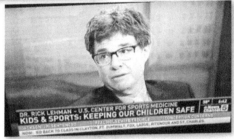
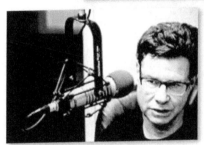
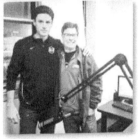
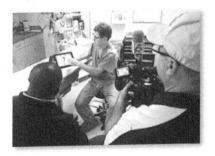

Top to bottom, left to right: in the studio hanging with the Fox 2 weathermen, the Charlie Tuna show broadcasting from a St. Louis area Schnucks, KSDK report on keeping kids safe in sports; on the radio for the Dr. Rick show; waiting to interview Adnan Gabeljik for the Dr. Rick show, taping a segment for KSDK 5 in St. Louis.

Living and Loving Life – I don't take for granted the opportunities I've been afforded to enjoy music, sports, travel, fitness, and unique life experiences and I'm looking forward to many more such chances ahead. Life is about the long-game and it is my hope that we raise athletes who get to enjoy it as such by taking better care of them!

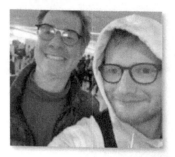
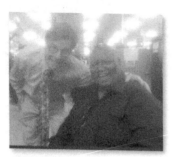

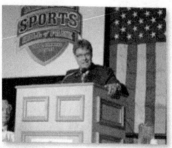

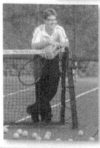
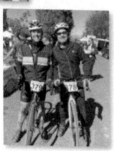

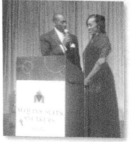

Top to bottom, left to right: off to an Antarctica trip with Ed Sheeran—December 2019; hanging with Charles Glenn before he sings the National Anthem for the St. Louis Blues; accepting my induction into the Missouri Sports Hall of Fame; hanging on the tennis courts for a St. Louis Business Journal piece; enjoying a bike race with Ryan Barber; supporting my friend Jackie as her brother Al Joyner presents an award to her.

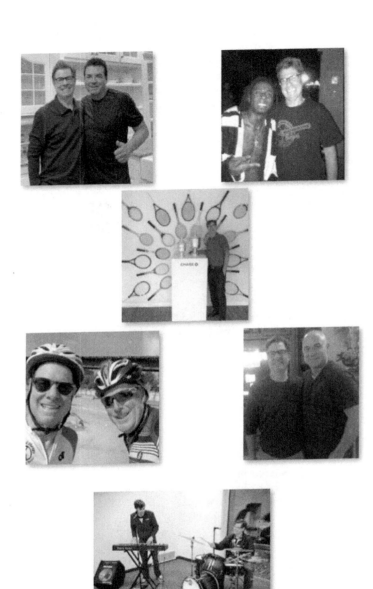

Top to bottom, left to right: enjoying time with my friend John (Papa John) Schnatter; hanging out with Lil Wayne at a concert; in awe of the trophy room at the U.S. Open— 2019; taking in a bike ride with my friend, Joe Dolan; supporting Andre Agassi at his "Play for Luke" charity event; making music with Mark Justice.

Practice and Patients — I love what I do. I love the people I work with and the experiences we have in helping others. Those others become friends . . . and families . . . *for life* and many of them visit with their families. I'm grateful to have lifelong relationships with these special people in my life.

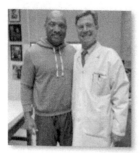
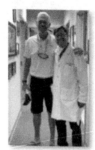
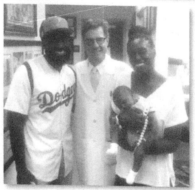
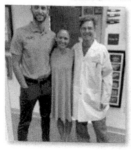
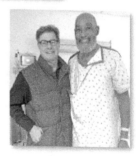

Top to bottom, left to right: visiting with NFL Hall-of-Famer Aeneas Williams, golfer Jay Delson dropped by; I loved meeting Dawn Harper Nelson and Alonzo Nelson's daughter Harper; U.S. Center for Sports Medicine visitors Gabby and Demos Dalton; amazed at my friend Olympic gold-medalist Greg Foster's recovery from heart surgery.

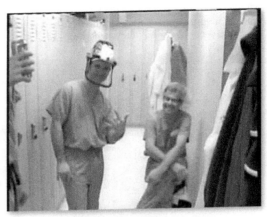

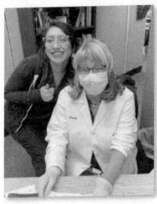

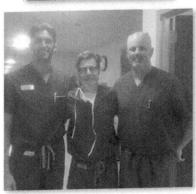

Top to bottom: in the locker-room before surgery; Eddy and Carla (my essential right hand) keep things running at the office; feeling short between my colleagues Dalton Demos and David Thomas.

Sports Stories — Aiding them as a doctor, witnessing them as a fan, or sharing them with a friend, from the training center to the trophy room, nothing brings adrenaline like a good sports story, and I'm grateful to have enjoyed many

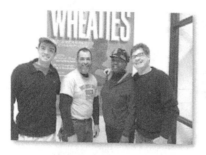

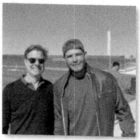

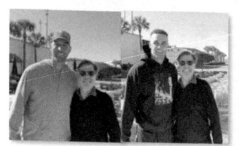

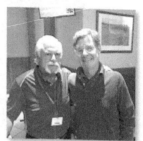

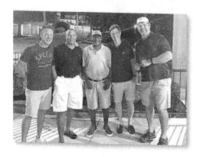

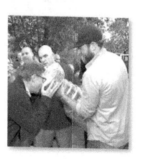

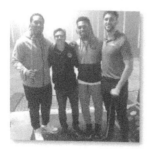

Top to bottom, left to right: at the Jackie Joyner-Kersee Community Center; Yadier Molina, then Adam Wainwright, then Jack Flaherty and I at spring training in Jupiter, Florida—2020; enjoying a Cardinal game with Al Hrabosky—August 2019; time with the Maryville University Track Coaching Team including Head Coach Vince Bingham; Ryan O'Reilly lets me kiss the Stanley Cup with Chris Kerber nearby; Dalton Demos and I with Darrian and David Bass.

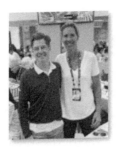
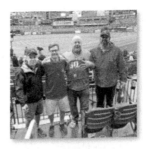
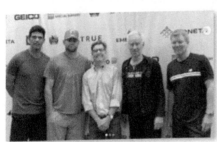
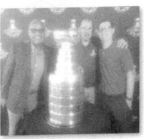
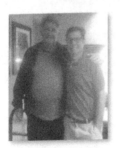
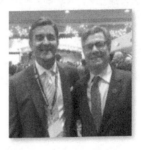
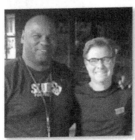
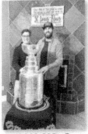

Top to bottom, left to right: with Brenda Schultz at the 2019 U.S. Open; enjoying an October 2019 Cardinal game with Mark LeGrand and Kevin and Tony Slaten; October 2018 with the greats—Andy Roddick, John McEnroe, Jim Courier, and Mark Philippoussis; KMOX's Mike Claiborne and Chris Kerber pose with me with the Stanley Cup; Mike Shannon and I at Busch Stadium, my friend Frank Cusumano gets inducted into the Missouri Sports Hall of Fame; enjoying time with Coach Mike Jones; Ryan O'Reilly and I with the Stanley Cup.

Family and Friends – This is who makes it all worthwhile; those pictured here and those not with whom I've shared my life; parents, siblings, wife, children, colleagues and patients who become lifelong friends, and so many more. They're not all in these pages, but they're all in my heart.

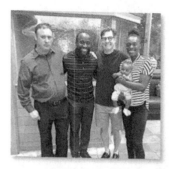
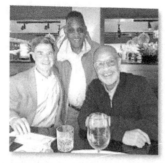

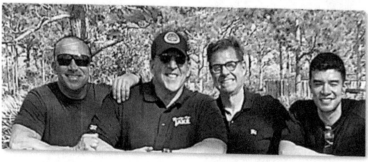

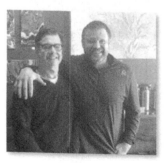
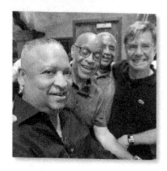

Top to bottom, left to right: Surf and Sirloin dinner with Dawn Harper Nelson, Alonzo Nelson, and daughter Harper; a night with Charlie Tuna and Mike Claiborne; my son Cameron and I enjoy time at Pine Creek Hunting Club with Jordan Zimmerman and Jake (Body by Jake) Steinfeld; coffee with my friend, retired NHL enforcer Tony Twist; guys' night with Reggie Smith, Mike Claiborne, and Darryl Bills.

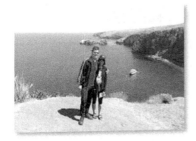
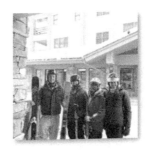
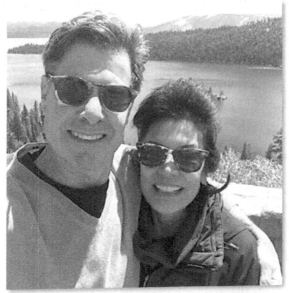
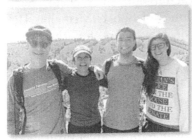
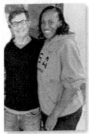

Top to bottom, left to right: traveling with my wife (and co-author) Michele Koo in California, the whole family—Cameron, Alex, Michele, and Sydney—on a Deer Valley, Utah ski trip in 2019; Doctors and spouses Dr. Richard C. Lehman and Dr. Michele Koo at Lake Tahoe; Michele and I enjoy a birthday weekend with two of our three children, Cameron and Alex; with my good friend Jackie Joyner-Kersee at the start of this book journey.

About the Author

DR. RICHARD C. LEHMAN is an orthopedic surgeon licensed in Missouri and California. He treats track and field athletes worldwide, as well as collegiate and professional athletes across America, and he specializes in rehabilitation of knee, shoulder, and elbow.

Dr. Lehman grew up in Miami, Florida. He studied medicine at the University of Miami and concluded his medical training at Washington University in St. Louis and the University of Pennsylvania. He has been the team physician for the Florida Panthers, Tampa Bay Lightning, and St. Louis Blues, has been a consulting physician for UCLA Track and Field, and has covered four Olympic Games, as well as seven Track and Field World Championships. He was inducted into the St. Louis Sports Hall of Fame and the Missouri Sports Hall of Fame in 2012. Among his surgical achievements, he has revolutionized cartilage regeneration and has written and lectured extensively on the subject. He has been published broadly in orthopedic and sports medicine literature and is the author of three books on tennis injuries.

Dr. Lehman formerly served on the Board of Directors of the Jackie Joyner-Kersee Foundation and is the current the medical director of Webster Surgery Center and the U.S. Center for Sports Medicine. He has served on the Board of Governors for the National Hockey League and sits on the St. Louis Sports Commission.

When not building his surgical practice, Dr. Lehman consults for several medical programs and is a proud husband, father, dog-owner, and lover of sports of all kinds. He also enjoys travel, nature, adventure, and rap.

For more information or to book an event, please contact RaiseAthleteIQ@gmail.com.

CURRICULUM VITAE

Richard C. Lehman
Missouri Sports Hall of Fame Inductee 2012
St. Louis Sports Hall of Fame Inductee 2012

Office:
U.S. Center for Sports Medicine
333 S. Kirkwood Road, Suite 200
St. Louis, Missouri 63122

Licensure and Certification Specifics:

- Licensure:
  - Missouri   R5B91
  - California   G5015
- Certification:
  - American Board of Orthopedic Surgeons, July 8, 1988- December 31, 1998
  - American Board of Orthopedic Surgeons, January 1, 1999- December 31, 2008, Re-certified American Board of Orthopedic Surgeons, January 1, 2009 December 31, 2018
  - Orthopedic subspecialty Certification in Sports Medicine, November 11, 2007- December 31, 2017
  - Carticel Sanofi Biosurgery Training Certificate for Implantation, October 15, 2013
  - Combined American Board of Orthopedic Surgery Certification & Subspecialty Certification in Sports Medicine, 2018-2028

Undergraduate Education:

- University of Minnesota, 1972-1976
- B.A. Major, Psychology
- B.A. Minor, Chemistry

Graduate Education:

- University of Miami School of Medicine, 1980, M.D. Degree

Post Graduate Education & Special Training

- Internship Barnes Hospital/Washington University, St. Louis, Missouri, 1981
- Orthopedic Surgery Residency Barnes Hospital/Washington University, St. Louis, Missouri, 1981-1985
- Sports Medicine Fellowship, University of Pennsylvania, Philadelphia, Pennsylvania, 1985-1986

Academic or Other Teaching Assignments:

- Chief Instructor (Orthopedic Curriculum) Washington University School of Physical Therapy and Irene Walter Johnson Institute of Rehabilitation, 1984, 1985
- Research Assistant Professor, Washington Univ. School of Medicine. Program in Physical Therapy and Irene Walter Johnson Institute of Rehabilitation, 1986 – 1992
- Orthopedic Peer Review Committee, Prudential Insurance Company of America, 1989

Hospital Appointments:

- Des Peres Hospital
- St. Clare Hospital
- Webster Surgical Center

Medical or Civic Appointments:

- Team Physician, U.S. Nationals Track and Field 2013
- Board of Directors, St. Louis Sports Commission
- Committee Member, National Multiple Sclerosis Society, Gateway Area Chapter
- Medical Director, U.S. Center for Sports Medicine
- Medical Director, Webster Surgery Center
- Team Physician, St. Louis Tennis Aces
- Consulting Physician, UCLA Track & Field
- Board of Governors, National Hockey League
- Missouri Athletic Association, Sports Medicine Hall of Fame Award
- Board Member, Dwight Davis Tennis Center
- Board of Directors, Jackie Joyner-Kersee Youth Foundation

- Board of Directors, General Resonance
- Inductee, Missouri Sports Hall of Fame Class 2012
- Medical Director, State Games of America
- Team Physician, Fox High School
- Team Physician, Maryville College
- Team Physician, Mehlville High School
- Team Physician, Missouri Baptist College
- Team Physician, Philadelphia Flyers Hockey Franchise
- Team Physician, St. Louis Blues Hockey Franchise
- Team Physician, St. Louis Sting Hockey Franchise
- Team Physician, United States Power Lifting
- Team Physician, United States Swimming
- Team Physician, United States Tennis Davis Cup Team
- Medical Advisory Board, American Red Cross
- Medical Director, HealthSouth Rehabilitation
- Medical Director, Tampa Bay Lightning

Educational Honors:
- Phi Beta Kappa, University of Minnesota, 1976
- Phi Kappa Phi, University of Minnesota, 1976
- Williams' Scholarship Award, University of Minnesota, 1973-1976
- Academic All American Tennis, 1973, 1974
- National Academic Award for Scholastic Athletes, Univ. of Minn., 1974-1976
- University of Miami Selected Exchange Student (6 students selected) 1980
- Lake Tahoe Fracture Clinic Selection, 1983
- Easter Orthopedic Cervical Spine Research Award, 1986

Scholarly Society Memberships (Previous and Current):
- American Academy of Orthopedic Surgeons
- American Board of Orthopedic Surgery
- American College of Sports Medicine
- American Medical Association
- Missouri State Medical Association
- St. Louis Arthroscopy Association
- St. Louis Metropolitan Medical Society

- The Society for Tennis Medicine & Science
- Southern Medical Association
- Southern Orthopedic Association
- Suffolk Academy of Medicine
- University of Pennsylvania Orthopedic Alumni

Athletic and Professional Awards:

- University of Minnesota, Varsity Tennis, 1972-1976.
- University of Minnesota, M-Award, 1973
- Williams' Scholarship, University of Minnesota, 1973, 1974, 1975, 1976
- Big Ten Conference Championships, 1973, 1974
- Missouri Athletic Trainers Association Sports Medicine Hall of Fame Award, 2006

Publications, Media Segments, and Studies:

Please contact our offices for a full current listing of all publications including more than eighty referred articles, non-referred articles, submitted articles, projects, or presentations. In addition, our offices can provide a full current listing of all traditional and non-traditional media features including more than fifty appearances across television, radio, newspapers, and web-based media resources and podcasts. Lastly, we are happy to provide an up-to-date listing of all past-conducted and in-process individual and joint studies.

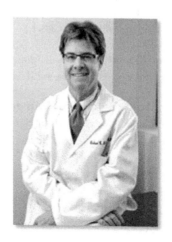

With Appreciation

First and foremost, I must thank my wife, Dr. Michele Koo. No matter how discouraged I was, or how much I wanted to give up, you never let me quit. You tracked down everything and everyone I needed to get this book to print. You were the driving force that got me through this project.

I'm grateful for the many friends, family, and community members who provided support, content, and insights. This list could be infinite, but I would specifically like to express my gratitude for: Dr. Torg, Ivory Crockett, Mike Keenan, Reggie Smith, Frank Cusumano, Louis Diguiseppe, Rob Campbell, Tony Twist, Nino Fennoy, Ken Dayley, Jay Harrington, Patrick Hulliung, and the Jenson family.

To Jackie and Bobby: we aren't just a team; we're family. I am honored to know you and grateful for your contributions, not just to this book, but to my life.

To my medical partners and colleagues, my life and practice are what they are because of you: Dr. Steven Stahle, Patrick Huck, Carla Droege, and the rest of *my* team.

And to my son Cameron who helped write these words, what a joy it was to create this with you. I am honored to be the father of you and both of your incredible sisters, Sydney and Alex.

Thank you all.

"While nobody asked for it, we have an opportunity for the ultimate athletic gift: a do-over. Let's not screw this up!"

Made in the USA
Las Vegas, NV
25 February 2021